Birth Book #2

8 Proven Ways to Have a Healthier Baby After Birth

(what studies show and many providers
never tell you about your baby's
first hour after birth)

By Sarah & Steve Blight

Birth Book (this book and other pregnancy books in this series) is not intended as medical advice (before pregnancy, during pregnancy, before birth, while giving birth, after birth or at any other time). *Birth Book (and other pregnancy books in this series)* is for educational, entertainment and informational purposes about pregnancy and about childbirth. Always consult a qualified medical or health professional during pregnancy for anything related to you and your pregnancy or your baby's health. The ideas, comments and suggestions contained in *Birth Book* (and other pregnancy books in this series) are not intended as a substitute for consulting a qualified physician during pregnancy or in birth. Nor should they ever be substituted for obtaining medical supervision regarding any activity, procedure, or suggestion that might affect your health before pregnancy, during pregnancy, before birth, in birth, after birth, or at any other time. Neither the author, contributors, nor the publishing company shall be liable or responsible for any loss, injury, or damage allegedly arising from any information or suggestion in *Birth Book (or other pregnancy books in this series)*. This book may contain affiliate links. That means some links in *Birth Book* may go to websites that compensate the authors, should you decide to buy anything from those sites. If you're still reading this, holy moly, you're probably the only one who ever will in the next hundred years. Congrats—we love that you're here & have a great day!

Kudos

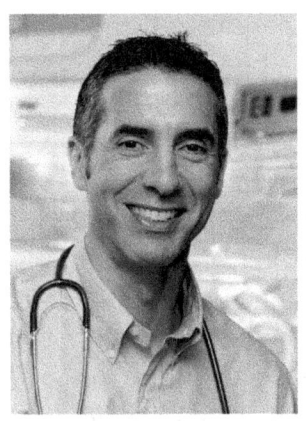

"Many expectant mothers don't know they can help improve their baby's health in that first hour after birth. The book is balanced, well-researched and easy to read. I have personally witnessed this "Golden Hour" for 30 years and have had the privilege of examining hundreds of thousands of babies in that first hour. This is an hour that can form our children for a lifetime. My daughter is due soon and I want her to read this book before she gives birth. If you're expecting a baby, get this book."

-Dr. Marc Belcastro (dad, director of NICU & Nurseries)

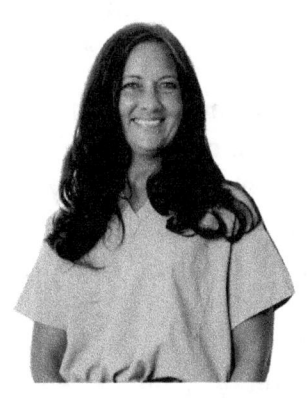

"As a mom of 4, former doula, and now OB/GYN, I believe your baby's health can be improved by reading this book. These new perspectives on the miraculous physiology at the moment of birth will redefine the maternity standard of care across all birth settings. Women preparing for birth, and those who assist them, will equally benefit from the wisdom expressed in Birth Book #2. Read this book!"

-Dr. Tami Michele (mom of 4, OB/GYN, & former doula)

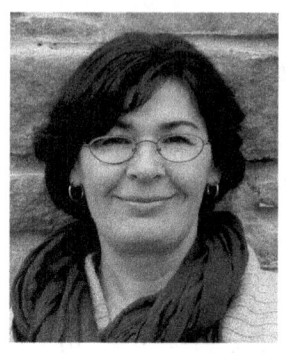

"The book that every parent-to-be and birth professional have been waiting for! In a simple but professional way, Sarah & Steve present evidence based information that your care provider will probably never share with you. Parenting decisions start when babies are still in the womb. You will learn everything about those precious hours after the birth of your baby, so you can make informed decisions for your family. I'm a certified birth doula and a certified childbirth educator. This book is a reliable source of information and I do highly recommend it to all my clients."

-Odile Penet (doula, childbirth educator)

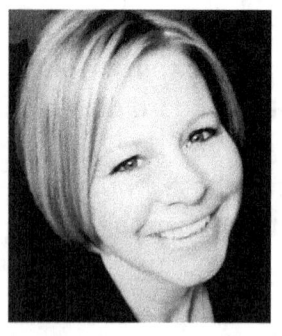

"Birth Book #2 is a real eye opener and a helpful tool for parents who want to have an optimal, immediate bonding experience with their baby. We already know that pregnancy and birth is a true miracle and now learn how those first few hours of the baby's life can be a continuation of that miracle, fostered with simple tools, resulting in lifelong benefits for parents and baby!

-Mary Ward (mom of 1)

Your Free Gift

To say a hugemongo "thank you" to our fabulous, loyal readers for buying this book, we wanted to give you a FREE chapter from another book!

We know you'll love it because lots of other mamas have shared how helpful it's been on their journey to the MotherLand.

The chapter comes from Birth Book #1 and is called, "How to Be Relaxed, Calm and Confident in Labor and Birth" with Dr. Bethany Hays (top OB/GYN and mom of 3). She'll most definitely inspire you and teach you how and why you're way more capable than you think you are!

Enjoy this chapter friends and thanks again for all your support!

You can download your FREE chapter by going here:

http://yourbabybooty.com/ybb/birthbook1-freechapter

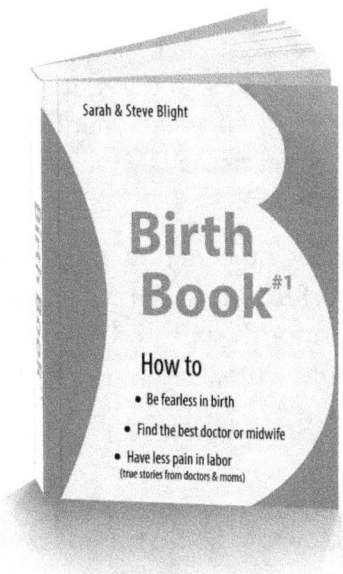

How this book will help you have a healthier baby

You've just given birth and you FINALLY get to see the sweet face that goes with those precious little limbs that have been kicking the stuff out of your bladder all those months. You're teary eyed and completely bewildered that your baby is finally here. You're parents! You and your hubby are on cloud nine. Baby is lying on your chest at last!

Did you know your baby's first 60 minutes after birth are called "The Golden Hour?"

Dr. Michele Odent, a famous Ob/Gyn says, *"The hour following birth is undoubtedly one of the most critical phases in the life of human beings."*

Our babies have to complete at least a dozen miracles in their first hour after birth to be healthy.

This is the most important hour of their lives, and yet, it's the most overlooked part of the whole pregnancy and childbirth shabang. Everything your baby has to miraculously (and instantly) start doing *after birth* is taken for granted.

It's taken for granted because we have no clue how much has to happen behind the scenes in our perfect, little, miracle baby's body. All we see is our baby's soft, smooth skin, and sweet little suckling lips, and tiny, tiny fingers with cuticles that are itty bitty.

We see perfection.

But mama, there is soo much more.

The time right after we meet our baby for the first time is sweet. Oh so sweet.

But are we missing out on doing the things that are scientifically proven to help our babies be as healthy as they can be? Are we missing out on forming those important first bonds of trust that will actually help our baby successfully adapt to the world outside the womb and that'll last forever?

We are watching them transition without participating. And the fact is, we could easily be helping them along.

Isn't that crazy?

Why just sit and watch when science has proven how we can help our baby do their miracle of transitioning to "life after the womb" AND improve their health at the same time?

The best medical research centers in the world have studies and evidence showing (which you'll see in the book) how we can "measurably improve" our baby's health after birth (and maybe even for life). The best part ...these things are super easy to do! Anyone can give their baby these health benefits (even if you've had a c-section).

What if ...

... your birth class and your provider just came out and said ... "Ok, here's how we can improve your baby's health, BIG TIME, in the first hour after they're born and maybe even for the rest of their lives. Let's walk through your options and look at the research evidence so you can understand your opportunity to give your baby a bunch of 'clinically measurable' and significant health improvements."

Since we've never heard of that happening for any mom, we wanted to write the book that did it for you. And make it easy to read.

That's why we wrote this book for you. To make sure you know how easily you can help your baby during the most important hour of their life, right when they need your help most.

It's true, many birth classes, providers and hospitals never tell you WHAT these easy things are that you can do. And they never teach you HOW to do them.

During that first hour, your baby has to:

1. Inflate their lungs to take their first breath and exchange oxygen for the first time - that's why you want to hear them cry.

2. Circulate blood to all their capillaries - that's why you want to see them "pink-up" in color.

3. Automatically close their heart's *ductus arteriosus* blood vessel, so they can grow-up with a healthy heart.

4. Use their own liver for the very first time, so they can metabolize fat stores for energy and growth.

5. Jumpstart their immune system for the first time in a big way, so they can fight off bacteria and disease with antibody packed breast milk and skin to skin contact.

6. Use their gastrointestinal system for the very first time, so they can digest nutrients and grow.

7. Use their skin to start regulating their own body temperature for the first time.

8. Instantly figure out the "suck, suck, swallow, breathe" pattern to successfully get all the nutrients from breastfeeding.

9. Adjust neurologically to gravity, which their brains, bodies and organs have never had to deal with before.

10. Last but not least ... your baby's heart! Your baby's heart has to start pumping oxygen to all their vital organs, organs which are just now "turning on" and working for the very first time (your placenta did all the work for those organs before birth).

And to think all this is just happening while you're wiping away the tears from your eyes, in disbelief that you're finally meeting your sweet bundle of joy.

Here's the truth ... while you can't control some things in birth, you do have 100% control over your precious baby getting these scientifically proven benefits that give them better health. You just need to know what they are and how to get them for your baby.

After reading this book, you'll know what these benefits are and how to get them for your baby. This book will teach you the medically proven ways to help your baby transition to life outside the womb during that critical first hour of life, their golden hour.

You'll learn how to:

✓ Help your baby take their first breath, breathe easier and lessen the chance of respiratory distress (one of the most common newborn health issues)
✓ Make breastfeeding happen more easily
✓ Optimize your baby's iron stores, which is important for healthy brain development
✓ Get your baby more oxygen for healthier brain functioning
✓ Help your baby's vital organs receive more oxygen, which is the most important thing they need when they start working for the first time

- ✓ Protect your baby against life-threatening vitamin k deficiency bleeding
- ✓ Boost your baby's immune system to fight off bacteria and infection
- ✓ Help your baby's body get more of the uber important stem cells

You'll see the proven research evidence that back up these benefits (from the best medical research centers in the world).

You'll learn from several of the country's best doctors, midwives and a leading evidence-based-birth researcher. They'll teach you WHAT these benefits are, HOW to give them to your baby and HOW to get them in whatever birth environment you decide is best for you (hospital, birth center or home birth).

You'll walk away feeling even more excited because you'll be more equipped to meet your little bundle of joy. And you'll feel better knowing how you can give your baby a jumpstart on their life!

One of the doctors we interviewed told us that his wife said ... "*I wish I would have known about this stuff when we had our two kids.*"

And to make it easy for you, we've created simple action steps at the end of each chapter. This helps you know exactly what to do and how to do it. We've created printable downloads that summarize and list the research evidence in the book, so you can take these bad boys with you to your appointments. And we've included exact scripts you can use when talking about these things with your provider, so you can feel better during your appointments.

Are you ready to dive in and learn what a rock star your baby is and how you can help improve your little rock star's health?

Let's hit it!

Sarah Stern

Table of Contents

respiratory problems during birth. And he delves into what hospitals and practices do with parents, which give them the best birth outcomes. Dr. Jain knows how to help babies stay healthy (he's in charge of a NICU).

Chapter 3 **"How Skin to Skin Can Improve Your Baby's Health & Double Your Breastfeeding Success" -with Barbara Harper, RN, Midwife, Birth Educator, Founder of Waterbirth International, Mom of 3**

The health benefits of skin to skin for both baby and mama are off the charts. You'll learn what these benefits are, how they can improve your baby's health and why you'll have a better bond with your baby forever (hint- your brain changes). You'll also see the proven research evidence backing up the benefits of skin to skin.

Since most hospitals don't usually do skin to skin, we show you how you can still get it wherever you decide to give birth, give you exact scripts you can use with your provider and even printouts you can easily take to your appointments outlining all the benefits and research evidence.

You'll also hear a story about why one mom is convinced that doing skin to skin helped save her baby who was born at 26 weeks.

Chapter 4 **"How to Get Skin to Skin With Your Baby During a C-Section" -with Mavis Schorn, CNM, Associate Professor of Nursing at Vanderbilt University, Mom**

You can still have skin to skin with your baby after a c-section. Mavis Schorn, a certified nurse midwife at one of the country's top hospitals, and her team, have pioneered a way that improves c-sections for every mom and baby. She teaches you how you can have skin to skin with your baby after a c-section.

Chapter 5 **"How Waiting 2 Minutes Can Improve Your Baby's Health for Life" -with Dr. Sarah Buckley, MD, Author, Mom of 4**

Waiting two minutes might give your baby the single most critical health boost they ever receive. It reduces the risk of anemia, improves brain development, helps their vital organs function better, gives their heart, brain and bodies up to 33% more blood and more oxygen, and even gives them more stem cells (which could someday save their life).

Delayed cord clamping is backed by the best research evidence (which we'll show you) and suggested by the leading medical research centers of the world.

Since most hospitals don't usually do delayed cord clamping, we show you how you can still get it wherever you decide to give birth. You'll also get exact scripts you can use with your provider and printouts you can take to your appointments outlining all the benefits and proven medical evidence. You'll be all ready to go and completely prepared for your prenatal appointments.

Chapter 6 **"Should I Consider Cord Blood Banking?" -with Dr. Sarah Buckley, MD, Author, Mom of 4**

Cord Blood Banking can be confusing and feels intimidating when we're bombarded by all the advertisements. Finally, clarity on cord blood banking! Alongside Dr. Sarah Buckley, we explain all the facts and available research evidence. You'll learn why you might want to consider it (or not) and the nitty gritty details - how it actually works, how much it costs and if it could help your family. No more confusion and no more feeling intimidated ... phew!

Chapter 7 **"Does My Baby Need Eye Ointment Right After Birth?" -with Rebecca Dekker, PhD, RN, Mom of 3**

Top evidence based researcher, Rebecca Dekker, holds your hand and walks you through the evidence about that eye goop they put in babies' eyes after birth. Dr. Dekker covers why it's done, the history behind it, if it helps your baby and what to do if you don't want your baby to have it.

Chapter 8 **"How Vitamin K Can Save Your Baby After Birth. What's the Best Way to Give Vitamin K?" -with Dr. Robert Sidonio Jr., Pediatric Hematologist, Dad & Dr. Anna Morad, Director of Newborn Nursery, Pediatrician, Mom**

We called in the big guns to dispel misinformation about the vitamin k injection babies often receive at birth. Drs. Sidonio and Morad explain the research and real-life implications of the vitamin k deficiency babies are born with, so you can decide if the vitamin k injection, oral version or doing nothing at all is best for your baby. They've made it their professional and personal mission to arm parents with the best evidence based information as they make their decisions (because they've been realizing in their practice that parents are getting bad internet based info). So we're giving you the facts ma'am. Just the facts.

Resources & Where To Go From Here

About

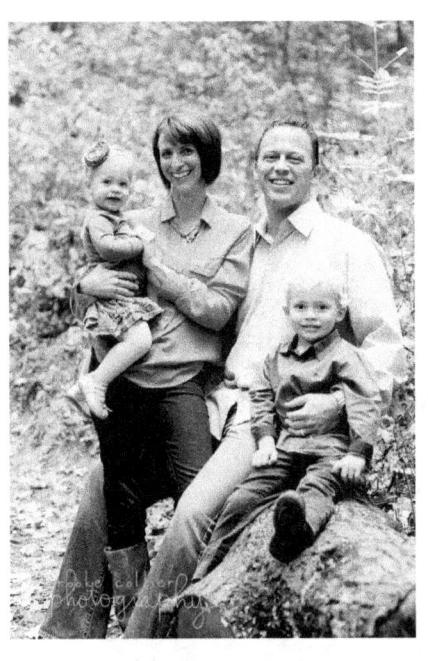

Hi, it's Sarah, we're so glad you're here ... congrats on being preggo or working on getting there!

After my first (of many) hormonal breakdowns in the middle of a baby superstore, I realized my overwhelming experience with baby registry and preparing for baby was common among new mamas. As I continued chattin' with new mamas and while trying to figure out what the heck to do for my own birth, I realized something else, most of my friends were not taught and didn't know how many safe (proven by medical research) options they had during pregnancy and birth—options that lead to easier, better and healthier outcomes for baby and mom-options that help us to feel intensely equipped and excited about birth.

I started having tons of friends, friends of friends, etc. ask me about everything I was learning from all my research ... and they were blown away by all the game-changing things they were *never taught* by their birth class or provider.

I had to do something.

So I brought the proven research from all the best and most respected people right to them.

I connected with hundreds of the top doctors, doulas, midwives, lactation consultants, fitness experts, renowned researchers, nutritionists and real moms and created a spot where they teach us all our options, in a relaxed, easy to understand, convenient and fun way.

There's no right way to birth a baby, but there's a right way for you.

If you want to learn the proven ways to have an easier labor and healthier birth, in a relaxed and stress free kinda way, then this Birth Book series was written for you!

If you like what you're reading, you'll love our site www.YourBabyBooty.com.

Or if you'd like to get an email when we release our next new book, just drop your email here: (http://yourbabybooty.com/ybb/future-books) & we'll let you know when it's hot off the presses. We're working on another new book now!

I (Sarah) am married to Steve and together we have two kids: our son born in a beautiful hospital birth who is now 4 (where does the time go?) and an equally amazing birth at home with our daughter (she's almost 2). We live up north in a state with lots of woods and beautiful lakes ... Michigan!

Chapter 1

How Your Silent Hormones Will Help You Birth a Healthier Baby (if you know how to let them)

with Dr. Sarah Buckley, MD, Author, Mom of 4

You don't need to be pregnant to know that hormones can take a sweet, funny, social butterfly of a woman and turn her into a raging, emotional, nutcase who is better left alone. We see hormones as "the culprit" – the culprit responsible for turning our emotions inside out and making us feel nasty, bloated, fat, and just downright ugly at times.

We think they're just another (one of the many) big pain in the arse side effects we have to deal with that make our lives way more emotional than they already are. And it's true. Sometimes they put us on a short fuse and make us feel a little wackadoodledo.

BUT, there's a secret.

A secret many doctors never teach their expecting mamas. A secret many of us never understand. It's a secret that actually helps us speed up labor, have a less painful childbirth and that literally turns us into superhero, supermoms.

And the secret is this...

Your hormones are THE secret sauce that will give you a smoother, faster, easier, less painful and healthier pregnancy, labor and birth.

Your hormones whisper to your body, guiding and directing it through your pregnancy and birth.

They prepare your mind to think and feel like a mom, even if you've never thought like a mom or felt like a mom before (and even if you've had anxiety about becoming a mom).

Your hormones are the reason why your body is so incredibly capable. And strong.

Your hormones are why YOU are so strong! And capable.

Yep, it' true, our hormones are our greatest asset and truly our best friend. But why? Like any best friend, sometimes they're a major pain. But they also save us in major, *major* ways.

Our hormones are most responsible for helping us (and our babies) get through the most important moments of our entire lives. And they work *really* well.

They're our constant, lifelong companions.

They usher us into puberty-oh the horror of those awkward years-and staying tried and true by our sides (okay more like in our sides) through our childbearing years. Then they give us one last big shove during our end of season, door-busting liquidation sale called "menopause."

The job of hormones, as you'll learn here, isn't to make our lives (or let's be honest, the lives of our partners) difficult.

Hormones actually make your pregnancy, your labor, your birth, your life and your baby's life way easier!

But only if you get out of their way and don't stop them from doing their thang.

Sounds like crazy talk you say?

Before you write me off, you've got to hear *why*. Then you'll get what I mean.

Enter Dr. Sarah Buckley.

We've found *the* leading expert on hormones, Dr. Sarah Buckley, to teach us how hormones make our lives easier, help us have less pain during labor, help speed up labor, protect our baby during labor, set us up for a lifelong bond with our babies and literally, like flipping a switch, turn us into mothers. Hormones are one of the big behind the scenes heroes that help our babies adapt and thrive as they start their life outside our womb.

There are tons of hormones at work in your pregnant body but the main ones are these guys:

-Oxytocin: a big one that bond baby and mama together. Also causes the uterus to contract and lots more which we'll delve into.

-Prolactin: this one's responsible for milk making, reduces our stress and turns on our mothering abilities.

-Beta-endorphin: all you need to know is "painkiller". This hormone helps us mamas get into the zone when we're in labor. Pretty ah-mazing.

-Epinephrine Norepinephrine: keeps mama alert as those beta endorphins are workin'.

-Progesterone: oh my, the jobs this hormone does are off the charts (literally), some of its duties are helping you get pregnant, slowing down your digestion when pregnant, and keeping things in line with your placenta.

-Estrogen: helps our uterus to grow, stimulates the oxytocin system, prepares our breasts for milk production (and lots more).

Dr. Buckley is a mom of 4 kids and a medical doctor with a specialty in obstetrics and hormones. She shares exactly how your and your baby's hormones work together, more seamlessly than a NASCAR pit crew team, to give you and your baby the best possible health.

Do you know how much better your life is because of your hormones?

A few things they do:

- Increase your chance of staying pregnant by helping implant the fertilized egg.
- Allow you to get baby out, during labor, easier and faster.
- Make your uterus grow so your baby has room to grow.
- Relieve pain during labor.
- Help breastfeeding happen easier last longer.
- Signal for your body to make breast milk.
- Help your baby's organs develop and strengthen their bone density.
- Literally turn on your "mothering" abilities so you can care for your baby (that's your 6th sense and mom intuition towards your kids).
- Gives you a bond with your baby that literally lasts forever.
- Help you stay relaxed and avoid being a stress fest.

These are just a few of the things our hormones do. How important is this list!? Yep. Hormones are the underappreciated BFFs for all their life-changing, behind the scenes work.

They get so little respect.

When you're feelin' "off," feelin' bloated, feel like munchin' on some chocolate covered pickles, or maybe you've already left this book 5 times to go pee ... those are signs that your hormones are doing *very* important things to help you and your baby!

So let's go.

We're about to learn how you can use your hormones to optimize your and your baby's health. Be prepared to have your mind blown at what is going on inside your incredible body!

***

"Oxytocin actually alters our brain & probably permanently changes our brain by 'turning on' the areas we need for mothering."

-Dr. Sarah Buckley

Sarah: Dr. Buckley, from all your experience as a mom and as a doctor, what are you most inspired to share with expectant moms and why?

Dr. Buckley: Our bodies are superbly designed for pregnancy, labor, birth and mothering! But that's not something you hear very much.

Often times, women go into labor and birth thinking their body won't work and their body will have to have technology [meaning the hospital actively doing something- hooking you up to machines, giving you medicine of some sort, doing a procedure, etc.] just to even go into labor and to make their babies safe.

We think our bodies are lemons. We think they won't work. Our bodies are not lemons.

Your body is not a lemon.

Your body is superbly designed for pregnancy, labor and birth. You can trust your body. The hormonal flow that automatically happens in your body helps make labor and birth happen as easily and efficiently as possible.

Your hormones are designed to enhance safety for mother and baby. There are many safety features naturally built-in to labor and birth. We're only now beginning to understand what all of these are.

Hormones are also designed for pleasure for both baby and mom. It might not sound "pleasurable" when you think about labor and birth, but the hormones of labor and birth actually activate the reward centers in your brain. Those reward centers help you remember the "in the moment feeling" you've had at birth, so at some point in the future you say to yourself ... *"wow, that was incredible! I could definitely do that again!"*

Sarah: You mentioned that science is discovering how much birth impacts us throughout the rest of our lives. What do you mean by that and how is that possible?

Dr. Buckley: We remember the births of our babies in great detail. We remember them for the rest of our lives. There was some research done by Penny Simkin and they discovered that women very accurately remember details about their birth decades and decades later. I just watched an interview with another childbirth researcher and she has women contact her, who are in their 60s, 70s, and 80s, who still want to talk about the "challenges" they had during their birth. Your birth will stay with you. It's a very defining moment.

A good birth is the investment of a lifetime.

Not only for our memories, but birth is designed to set up the optimal physiology for mother and baby. It's designed to make baby optimally prepared for life outside the womb.

We're beginning to understand that birth is not just a one-off process that happens once in life and is forgotten about. And what happens for the baby during labor and birth actually *optimizes* the baby's physiology for much improved health and probably for their entire life.

Sarah: Let's help moms understand the big picture of hormones in our bodies. A lot of us have these negative associations or stereotypical pregnancy associations with hormones, but you said hormones are actually here to make our lives (and our baby's lives) easier during pregnancy, labor and birth. Can you give us a big picture perspective of what hormones are?

Dr. Buckley: A hormone is a substance that's made in one part of the body and it has actions or effects in another part of the body. The most common childbirth hormone I'll talk about is called oxytocin.

Oxytocin is naturally made in our brain. Specifically, it's made in the pituitary system of our brain, which is in the middle layer (limbic). Once we make it, we release it within the brain. We also release it into our bloodstream. During labor, it travels in the bloodstream to our uterus. Oxytocin causes our uterus to contract. So whenever we talk about "labor contractions," we're talking about our uterine muscles tightening or contracting (for the reason of pushing baby out), which was caused by that oxytocin.

Oxytocin is released in pulses from the brain, which is why we have our rhythmic contractions during labor [the same Oxytocin pulse released from our brain makes its way through our blood and then arrives at our uterus, which then rhythmically contracts it. The pulsing happens so our bodies have time to rest between contractions and also helps our babies rest between contractions too].

Oxytocin does a lot of other things too. It's the "chilling out" hormone and has been called the "hormone of calm and connection."

Our brain releases more oxytocin during labor and birth than any other time of life.

So when we have these peaks of oxytocin during labor and birth, especially right after our baby is born, you get that BIG rush of happiness, calm and connection. An oxytocin high is a great feeling to have!

It also switches on the mother's instinctive behaviors (which is true in every mammal). It actually alters our brain and probably permanently changes our brain by "turning-on" the areas we need for mothering.

Research shows how these peaks of hormones during labor and birth actually shift the mother's brain, so she can optimally mother her baby.

Oxytocin is that alertness, contentment, feel-good-feeling and happiness we get, when thinking about our babies that helps us care for them. We also get flooded with oxytocin when we hear our babies cry.

But it's not just a feeling. It's Mother Nature's biological programming.

It's actually how babies survived, how moms survived and how the species survived. It happens for every mammalian mother and it's true for human mothers as well. The *processes* of labor and birth are really *designed* to give us a head start with our mothering.

Sarah: Is that why when I hear my baby cry, my breasts leak milk?

Dr. Buckley: Yes, that's exactly right! You release oxytocin in your brain, which gives you all the alertness, empathy and reward feelings, but then it also comes down into your blood stream and actually causes a contraction in the muscle cells aligning your milk ducts. The milk ducts contract up and release the milk. That's the letdown reflex you're talking about. It happens both in your brain and in your body.

Sarah: That's incredible! To understand how hormones can make our lives so much easier, let's start by understanding where hormones come from and how they work?

Dr. Buckley: Hormones are generally made in our brains. They have effects within our brains and effects within our body. Oxytocin causes the contractions of labor and birth, the letdown reflex during breastfeeding. It actually causes your orgasm too!

It's the "sexual hormone" that flows during sexual activity. As it's released into the body, it's also released into the brain causing calm and connection. It's been called the "hormone of monogamy," because it causes bonding between men and women after sex. That's true for other monogamous species too.

It's also been called the "cuddle hormone" and of course the "mothering hormone" for the mothering behaviors we've talked about. So it's a whole package of things that happen when we make love, when we make babies, when we have a baby, when we breastfeed our baby, when we interact with our babies, etc.

Sarah: You've led into my next question: what's the big deal about hormones? You've already talked about oxytocin, but what about the other hormones, why do they matter to us?

Dr. Buckley: Okay. So using oxytocin as an example, it matters because Mother Nature's superb design gives us these peaks of oxytocin that optimize the efficiency of labor and birth. Hormones give us pain relief during contractions and they particularly optimize the efficiency of the pushing stage. They get us ready and make sure we're ready to push our baby out.

You get a big surge of oxytocin near the end of your labor. That surge gives you a big contraction, which helps your baby to be born quickly and easily.

And this is amazing ... after the birth, you get a ten times higher oxytocin surge than you ever had during labor and birth. The reason why this big surge is amazing, is because it's specifically designed to bond you to your baby.

Dr. Michel Odent, a world leading French OB/GYN, calls it *"the beginning of a great love affair."*

That oxytocin surge after birth is the biggest your brain will ever produce.

GOOD TO KNOW...

Think about this for a second: This is the biggest spike in oxytocin you'll ever experience in your life. You'll never have a surge like that again in your entire life and it's designed to bond you to your baby in deep, deep, love! How cool is that? I mean seriously, you can't write a better script for unconditional love.

You're chemically bonded to your baby. That means your brain, your heart, your entire being falls in love with your child. It lasts forever.

That's why they say there is nothing stronger than a mom's love for her child. Nobody experiences this chemical bond except the baby and mom (dad also has hormone boosts, but it's not anywhere close to the amount mom gets).

Have you heard of moms who instantly get super-woman strength to literally pick up a car to rescue their baby from danger? This is WHY and HOW it happens. Our brain floods our blood with these hormones (natural chemicals), which fuel our muscles with bursts of super-human strength, courage, etc. Those stories are real. It happens. It's science. It's part of our amazing physiology that helps protect our babies.

I don't know about you, but this floors me with awesomeness. Hormones help us have superwoman-like capabilities that we never tapped into, before becoming a mom.

***

Dr. Buckley: So your hormones will actively make mothering easier for you. Oxytocin has "the star role" you could say, because it helps so much throughout pregnancy, labor and birth, has a natural pain relieving quality and helps breastfeeding happen easier.

While we're breastfeeding our babies, we're getting some oxytocin, which rewards us, which makes us calm and connected, which increases our bond with our baby, makes us feel good, and actually helps improve the flow of all the other hormones.

So that's oxytocin...it's been the focus of a huge amount of research in recent years because it is the catalyst for so many positive things to happen for moms and babies.

Some of the other hormones that I write and speak about, beta-endorphins, adrenaline (also called epinephrine) and prolactin, are in more detail in my e-book *"Ecstatic Birth: Nature's Hormonal Blueprint for Labor"* at SarahBuckley.com. I recommend you look at that if you're interested to find out even more details about hormones.

Let's talk about the second hormone called beta-endorphin. Beta-endorphin, like oxytocin, stimulates our reward centers. And it also acts as a natural painkiller, so it's every mama's best friend in labor. And the further along you are in labor, the more beta-endorphins help you deal with stress and pain. It also pulls you into this altered state of consciousness. Do you remember that in your labor, Sarah?

Sarah: Yes, I do...I was totally in my zone. I've heard people talk about being in the zone, but never experienced it myself until my first birth. Hours felt like seconds, I don't remember anyone coming in or out, all I remember was my eyes being closed and I was completely focused and aware of what my body was doing and needed to do. It was an incredible feeling! I wish I could always be that focused, I would get so much done!!

Dr. Buckley: Naturally laboring and birthing women enter this altered state of consciousness; some people say it's "going to labor land." Some people share a Native American understanding that says, *"A laboring woman goes out to the stars to collect the soul of her baby and bring it back."*

That's exactly what is happening in labor. You're entering this altered state. It's human chemistry. It's science. It's physiology. You get this natural pain relief. It takes you into this state of transcendence, where you can transcend the stress and pain of labor.

It helps you follow your new mom instincts.

It's the hormone that helps your body know what it wants to do and do what it needs to do. If those hormones flow, you don't care what other people think, what they say, or what other people want of you. You're in this state where you can be very direct about what you want and need, which is so important in labor, because that's how you get all of your needs get met.

Getting ALL of your needs met, like being able to get into the laboring and birthing positions that feel most comfortable for you, to only have the people you want to have in the room with you, to be comfortable in the place you want to be laboring and birthing in. All of those increase the chances that your birth will go smoothly and easily.

Sarah: You're right, for me, I call it getting in my zone, but I really love the American Indian analogy. I'll have to admit, before birth, I probably would have said that sounded a little "woo woo" or "out there" to me, but after two births … I think it's right on. It's true. Whatever your experience, you just go to a place that you've never been to before, to bring your baby into this world.

You quoted a Dutch obstetrical professor in your book, who said … *"Spontaneous labor in a normal woman is an event marked by processes that are so complicated and so perfectly attuned to*

each other that any interference will only detract from the optimal character."

What does that mean and can you give us an example?

Dr. Buckley: Sure, as I've said, we're only really *beginning* to understand the whole complex orchestration of how hormones interact with each other during labor and birth. I love how he says, *"perfectly attuned."*

Your hormones are perfectly attuned with your babies.

A great example showing how hormones are perfectly attuned is the hormone epinephrine-norepinephrine. When a woman is naturally going through her labor, levels of this hormone gradually increase. She reaches high levels of epinephrine-norepinephrine toward the end of labor.

That's really important because she's in this altered state of consciousness, which is hugely beneficial to her, but she also needs to be alert.

For millions of years, mothers have given birth out in the wild, and it was a jungle out there. You never knew what animal or predator was around the corner, so going off into "labor land" might not benefit your baby if you weren't alert to the presence of danger.

Women who've already labored might remember this too … you're in this altered state of consciousness, but your hyper vigilant senses are also locked in. You're really sensitive to anything and everything going on around you. You're aware of *any* suggestion of danger. It's an extraordinarily unusual hormonal situation.

Here's a common example … let's say you're laboring in a hospital and you hear an unfamiliar voice all the way out in the corridor suggesting "something" about you, your baby, or your birth.

You're instantly fixated on whatever was just said. You're very alert to that.

So these natural hormones work as they gradually increase in strength, but if you feel frightened, scared or nervous, for whatever reason, during labor, or you don't have the basic requirements you want and need for labor, your brain will instantly release a different combination of hormones that chemically shut down your labor.

Your brain instinctively wants to protect your baby. So your body will actually start protecting your baby by shutting labor down.

All mammals need to feel private and safe and unobserved in labor. Every animal in the world needs to feel private, safe, and for any of you who've had animals under your care (maybe you've grown up on a farm, you've seen your domestic animals give birth, or even in the zoo), you know the caregiver's focus is on providing privacy and protection for that animal.

You want to get out of the way of that animal. You don't want to let her know you're there. You may even hide because your presence will interfere with the birth process for that animal. That's true for human mothers as well.

So if you were laboring, you'd be in tune to everything around you. While looking around, and if you had any slight sense of danger, you'd get an early elevation of these hormones. You'd get a spike of epinephrine-norepinephrine.

I call it the "saber-tooth tiger effect." Back in the jungle, if a woman was giving birth in the water and a saber-tooth tiger appears, the surge of these hormones would turn labor off. They would inhibit her contractions and shift her blood supply away from her uterus towards her major muscle groups.

If that were you laboring, your major muscle groups would get more blood so you could "fight" your way to safety or "flight" your way to safety. That's exactly what your body's "fight or flight" response is and how it works.

In doing so, blood shifts away from your uterus and baby.

This is why it's so important for us to feel safe and unobserved, because if we don't, we may have a surge of epinephrine-norepinephrine. Not only will our labor slow down, but our baby could potentially be deprived of blood and oxygen.

This explains what happens to women in hospitals when we don't provide conditions in the hospital where they feel private, safe and unobserved. We put them in a room with a bunch of strangers coming in and out of an unlocked revolving door. No other animal could give birth in that situation. It's ridiculous that we do that to laboring women. No wonder the reason most women need intervention is because their labor slows down. No wonder their babies may have a lack of blood and oxygen, which we call "fetal distress." We're not giving women the basic requirements they need and we end up with a lot of intervention necessary.

Our basic physiology hasn't changed in millions of years.

We still have those same requirements. This explains why women who use a doula during their hospital birth having lower interventions needs, because the doula helps them feel private, safe, and unobserved. It also explains why women who labor and birth at home have a much lower need for intervention.

Something else about the epinephrine-norepinephrine hormone I'd like to share, which is really important for the baby is when the baby gets towards that end of labor, the baby's head is low in the mother's birth canal, and pressure on the baby's head causes a surge of these hormones for the baby. That's called a catecholamine surge.

These hormones are for the baby. This hormone surge protects your baby. It protects your baby at that most intense time in labor, when your contractions are long, strong, and close together. Each time the uterus contracts, it deprives the baby of blood and oxygen to some extent.

But your baby is perfectly adapted to that. A healthy baby has no problems with that part of labor. The catecholamine surge protects the baby's brain from those long and close together contractions. It ensures there is always a good blood supply to the heart and the brain, which are the paths of the body that will need the blood and oxygen. It also begins to prepare the baby for life outside the womb, so it actually starts to prepare your baby for their first breath.

Your baby's lung surfactant increases, which is a lung lubricant. This will help ease the flow of air into the baby's lungs, it opens up the airways after birth. It also increases lung elasticity, and at the same time, the surge of catecholamines increases the baby's metabolic fuel, so the baby can have a good blood glucose level and have good metabolic fuels for that period after birth until their mother's milk supply comes in. It also begins the baby's process of generating their own heat or temperature; so it increases the baby's thermogenesis.

We can also see how important these hormones are for the newborn baby. The catecholamine surge also makes the baby wide-eyed and alert. So when you see those pictures of newborn babies who are really wide-eyed and alert, that means they've got a good surge of catecholamine hormones.

When you look at cesarean babies, often they have breathing difficulties. They tend to have low blood sugar. They tend to have poor temperature control, and all of these things can be explained because the cesarean baby, particularly the elective cesarean baby – the baby born by a scheduled C-section – doesn't have a surge of these hormones.

Sarah: So that catecholamine surge happens with labor?

Dr. Buckley: Yes.

Sarah: Okay. Let's talk about prolactin. Explain to us what that hormone is all about.

Dr. Buckley: Sure. These 4 hormones that we've been talking about, I call them the ecstatic hormones of labor and birth, because they're all really feel good hormones and they all benefit mothers and babies during the adaptation to life after birth.

We've talked about oxytocin, the hormone of love. We've talked about beta-endorphin, which are the hormones of transcendence. We've talked about epinephrine-norepinephrine and adrenaline-noradrenaline, which I call the hormones of excitement, because they make mother and baby excited.

Our fourth ecstatic hormone is prolactin, the hormone of mothering.

It's a hormone that builds up. We release it and we produce it during pregnancy. All during pregnancy it's really softening our brains and switching us on to mothering behaviors.

You know how when you're pregnant, you have this heightened sensitivity to babies and even baby animals … you might see a cute little baby animal and get really teary during pregnancy? That's' prolactin! Prolactin is working on your brain to soften it and prepare you for mothering.

And like oxytocin, it's also a chill-out hormone. It reduces your levels of stress and reduces your susceptibility to stress during pregnancy, during labor, during breastfeeding. Prolactin reduces your stress hormone levels.

And it's also pro-lactation. It's the major hormone of breast milk synthesis. All during pregnancy, these levels are increasing in your brain, but it doesn't actually switch on the production of breast milk until after birth.

The reason is because another hormone that is in the placenta, progesterone, inhibits its breast milk-producing activity. So after you've given birth and the placenta has been born, then suddenly prolactin kicks in and begins to produce breast milk for you.

And we know that during labor and birth like the other ecstatic hormones, prolactin levels change. It goes down during labor and then suddenly surges in the moments after birth for several hours afterwards, which is perfectly timed to help the mother's brain adapt for optimally mothering her baby.

We also know that when the mom and baby are together, skin-to-skin after birth, the baby starts to stimulate the mother's breast, the baby will massage the mother's breast, and then eventually suckle, and all of those activities stimulate prolactin release as well.

All of this helps to set up the mother's prolactin system for a really good milk production for the baby.

Sarah: Our bodies are seriously incredible! Our hormones are like a symphony, working together smoothly towards a healthy pregnancy and birth.

Let's put it all together for the mamas (since it can get a little confusing), so they can see the progression. Let's take it from the top and go from pregnancy all the way through labor and childbirth … how are all of these hormones interacting with each other?

Dr. Buckley: Great idea! First, there are many, many hormones in pregnancy, labor, and birth. I'm just singling out those four. The other major hormone is estrogen, which is the female hormone that we produce at levels about a thousand times higher by the end of pregnancy.

Estrogen gives us some of those things that happen first in pregnancy and helps to mature our breasts for breast milk production. Estrogen is important because it actually stimulates the oxytocin system. High levels of estrogen increase our oxytocin receptor numbers, which make our bodies more sensitive to oxytocin.

During pregnancy, oxytocin is made in our brains and helps us adapt to maternity by switching on those instinctive mothering behaviors. It also makes us chilled out. It's a calm and connection hormone, and all the time during pregnancy, the oxytocin system is being "up-regulated," which is a technical term for saying it's becoming more active.

As we're getting more receptors, we're getting more sensitive overall. The actual amount of oxytocin in our brain increases dramatically just before labor and birth. The timing is perfect. Just before labor and birth, we have the most sensitivity we'll ever have to oxytocin because we have the most of those hormonal receptors. The receptor sits on the outside of the cell wall. The hormone binds to the receptor. Right where it binds to the receptor, it sends a message into the cell telling it to do something.

So with oxytocin, it travels from our brain, through our blood, and binds to the receptors on the outside of the mother's uterine muscle cells. When it binds, it sends a signal saying, "contract." That's how oxytocin is released from our brain and causes your uterine contractions.

You can see that it's not just the amount of oxytocin in her bloodstream that determines how efficient her contractions are, but also the number of receptors that she has. So when she has the most receptors as her labor begins, her body will be very sensitive to oxytocin- that's why she'll get the most efficiency and ease out of labor and birth.

One thing that commonly happens, that few of us recognize-if our body is not close to going into spontaneous labor on its own (naturally), then we'll have a lower number of oxytocin receptors. That's why inductions sometimes don't work.

You can't tell when women's bodies are ready to go into labor on their own. Some animals you can. Rats for example, rats go into labor on day 22. Every rat goes into labor on day 22.

Women don't all go into labor on the same day. 5% of women go into labor on their due date. The natural onset of labor can happen anywhere from 36 to 37 weeks to 42 weeks. So it's a really wide range. So when the woman is ready to go into labor herself, she'll be really exquisitely sensitive to oxytocin.

And if you wanted to give her the drug of pharmacological oxytocin (that's what Pitocin is, synthetic oxytocin), just a little drizzle of it, and suddenly, labor would kick in. But if she's weeks away from the natural onset of labor, or weeks away from when her body is naturally ready with all those receptor cells ready to go, you could give her all the Pitocin you like and labor won't happen. The reason is because she just does not have the sensitivity.

These changes also involve changes in the woman's cervix. If the woman's cervix is "ripe," as we call it, which is soft and open and short (which means baby will have the easiest time coming through the birth canal … cervix means "neck of the womb" in

Latin), then that probably means her oxytocin receptor numbers are getting towards optimal.

Sarah: So you're saying literally from the moment you become pregnant, all your hormones are working together with the goal of getting baby out smoothly and easily?

Dr. Buckley: Yes, that's exactly right. There was a famous midwife from Utah who said, *"It's ridiculous to put a length of time on labor, because labor actually lasts 9 months. It takes 9 months to give birth."*

Sarah: I bet our spouses would agree that our hormones are flowing for a lot longer than 9 months!

We've talked about how the hormones in our bodies help us in major ways … let's do some role playing so mamas can get an idea of what this really looks while giving birth.

Let's say it's really loud where I'm laboring (hospital, birth center or home) and you hear someone say something that distracts you. Maybe it's something that is 100% unrelated to what you're trying to focus on during labor (like someone talkin' smack to their significant other) something that just rubs you the wrong way, maybe it's someone talking too loudly or even being snippy for some reason … how does that affect my labor and why?

Dr. Buckley: Wherever you are laboring, you need to feel private, safe, and unobserved during labor. When a woman isn't feeling private, safe and unobserved, her adrenaline-noradrenaline hormone levels can go up, and that will usually turn off her labor like turning off a switch. It can even interfere with the blood supply to a uterus and baby.

The conditions we need to have a baby are very similar to the conditions we need to make a baby.

So we need to feel private, safe, and unobserved, otherwise, it's not going to work. The same energy that is required to get the baby in gets the baby out. Private, safe, and unobserved is really important. Was that your experience?

Sarah: Yes, thankfully I did have that with both my births. When Jackson was born, we had the best labor and delivery nurse who gave us our space and honestly, I barely noticed when she came in or out. I had a horrible postpartum nurse who was loud and really bossy and I ended up in tears with her. She was awful. I was thanking my lucky stars that she wasn't the labor and delivery nurse!

So what can mamas do to be private, safe and unobserved during birth?

Dr. Buckley: You want to think about this beforehand. Organize a situation where you'll feel as private, safe, and unobserved as possible. I mentioned before that many women will instinctively choose the smallest most private room they can. Having someone that can help you protect your space, like a doula or your own midwife, is really important! And you may even choose to not leave your own space, to have your baby at home.

Sarah: That's a great suggestion about the doula.

Let's say I'm laboring in the hospital and I'm not progressing. The nursing staff walks in and says ... *"You're not progressing, we'd like to start you on Pitocin"* (which is the synthetic oxytocin drug). How does that affect me? How does that affect my baby?

Isn't the synthetic hormone drug just like the hormone I naturally have in my body?

Dr. Buckley: The synthetic hormone is very different than your natural hormone. Remember when I talked about how your natural oxytocin is released from your brain and goes into your body AND into your brain at the same time?

Because your body's natural oxytocin goes into your brain, that's why you get the calming, connectedness, loving and pain relieving effects. Synthetic oxytocin does not go into your brain – it goes straight into your body.

You get the effects on the uterus with contractions, but Pitocin gives you none of those calming, loving, connectedness and pain relieving loving effects. If you've ever been induced, or been with someone who has, you know exactly what I'm talking about. It's not a good feeling.

The contractions with Pitocin are longer, stronger, and closer together than a woman would have with her own naturally produced oxytocin. Because the contractions are much more unpredictable, it can cause a lack of blood and oxygen supply to the baby. It can cause fetal distress.

We know this is true because every time you have a Pitocin drip, you have to have an IV, you have to have continuous fetal monitoring. I say to women, *"You know, if you are offered an intervention that requires monitoring, you know there is a risk to your baby."*

There is a risk to your baby with synthetic oxytocin (i.e.- Pitocin).

The other thing that we know is that using Pitocin for prolonged periods of time detrimentally affects the mother's own oxytocin system. We talked about receptors beforehand. When the mother has excessive exposure to oxytocin, her receptors do a very sensible thing, they reduce in numbers. It's called "down regulation". The mom's body tries to make sure that she doesn't get over stimulated from the Pitocin given. That means that her body becomes less sensitive to oxytocin in general.

After the birth, when she really needs a good surge of oxytocin to protect her from bleeding (her natural oxytocin surges after birth helping to preventing postpartum hemorrhage by causing her uterus to contract very strongly), her low receptor numbers prevent her body from effectively responding.

So we know that women who have synthetic oxytocin in labor are more likely to bleed after the birth and require extra doses of Pitocin after the birth.

Something else to ask, *"What are the effects on baby?"*

We know oxytocin is the hormone of connection. It sets moms up to be a mother, to be alert and rewarded. What does it do in the long term to have the baby exposed to these high levels of synthetic oxytocin, because it does cross into the baby's brain?

We know from animal studies it can actually interfere with their hormonal systems lifelong. We haven't known to think about that for human babies, so the chances are that there is some effect, but we don't really know what it is at the present time.

Sarah: That's good-to-know and think about before we're even offered Pitocin. You mentioned the private, safe, and unobserved place is important to keep labor going, what else can mamas do if their labor has petered out?

Dr. Buckley: As I said, the energy that got baby in can get baby out, so let's talk about other ways we can naturally produce oxytocin. Stimulating our breasts produces oxytocin. Sexual activity produces oxytocin. Making love will literally make oxytocin and someone actually used this as an alternative when her labor slowed down! We made sure they were private, safe and unobserved when they were "smooching" with their sweetheart! We've even had orgasms in the labor ward. That really gives you a surge of oxytocin.

Sarah: I can attest to some of that! With my second baby, whom I gave birth to 18 months ago, my contractions were slowing down and my midwife was on her way. Once she showed up, we thought, *"Alright, let's see if this is real labor"*, and so we did a little nipple stimulation, and the contractions instantly picked up. It was like turning on a switch, everything just sprang to life! So oxytocin was definitely going on behind the scenes, right?

[Mama. Make sure you talk to your provider about doing any of these natural ways to induce your own labor- things can happen in a hurry and you want to be prepared or have someone ready to help you!]

Dr. Buckley: Exactly! And it also happened for you Sarah because you had large number of oxytocin receptors active, because you naturally went into labor and birth. So your oxytocin system was as sensitive as it could have been.

Just like you said, a little bit, and suddenly everything kicked in.

Sarah: The next scenario is when I ask for an epidural. How does an epidural affect me, my baby and the symphony of hormones that we now know is going on?

Dr. Buckley: Great question! An epidural really is the most effective form of pain relief. And it can be fantastic for some women. The problem is it affects all of our aesthetic hormones and that can have detrimental effects for mom and baby.

For example, when you have an epidural in place, within a few minutes, your oxytocin level starts to go down, and it basically goes down all the way through your labor. That means labor can slow down, and often it does. Most women with an epidural end up needing a Pitocin drip to really get labor started again.

I talked a little bit about that the laboring mom gets a surge of oxytocin towards the end of labor that helps her give birth

44

efficiently. The woman with an epidural particularly misses out on that. That's really not so good because that means that she's less likely to be able to push her baby out by herself, and increases her risk of needing forceps or a vacuum to help give birth. Neither of those things are much fun for the mama or fun for the baby and can increase the risk of tears for example, so that's the problem with epidurals and oxytocin.

Epidurals also reduce beta-endorphins, which is that hormone that puts you out into labor land. So the woman with an epidural doesn't experience that altered state of consciousness that Mother Nature designs to help women labor easier.

I read a book, and it said that when the woman gets the epidural, she becomes chatty to her girlfriends and nice to her husband, and that's true. The reason why is because when you're in this altered state of consciousness, you're acting instinctively and you'll do exactly what you need to do for your baby to be born. When you have an epidural, you are not in that altered state and you're more normal, you could say.

Sarah: So what I hear you saying is that epidurals are a trade-off. You can get very effective pain relief (or close to it), but the cost is that it disrupts the normal "balance" of hormones.

Dr. Buckley: And I think epidurals are really well intentioned. The medical system comes up with a very effective option to reduce pain, and it works. Women who've had an epidural have been very satisfied with their pain relief, but that doesn't mean they have been satisfied with their overall experience of labor and birth. Pain relief is one part of the bigger picture.

And I'm not saying that if you've had an epidural, you're not going to be a good mom.

I am saying Mother Nature designed us to have these hormones running through our brain and body to optimize our start to

45

mothering. And so our brain's reward centers are triggered and meshed with our babies so we can enjoy mothering ... it might be that an epidural interferes with that on some level.

Sarah: I'm really glad you said that - that's a good distinction! This is why we're here. We're not here to suggest a specific decision mama should take, but to support mama in whatever she decides. We want to make sure mamas have ALL the info they need to make the best decision for them. We're here to talk about the most important information, that'll have the biggest impact on having a healthy birth, that many birth classes never even teach and providers never share, and in a lot of cases, don't even know themselves.

I can't tell you how many moms have told me they wish someone had shared this kind of information with them BEFORE their birth, because had they known it, they'd have made different decisions.

Ok, let's talk about c-sections because I know there are women who have either had c-sections in the past or might need a c-section for a medical reason. You mentioned a little bit about the impact of c-sections and the hormone interchange that happens between you and your baby. Can you talk more about that?

Scheduled Cesarean-Section (also called Elective C-Section)

Dr. Buckley: We have two different kinds of cesareans from a hormonal perspective; let's start by talking about a scheduled c-section or an elective c-section.

The mom misses out on that hormonal preparation and the baby misses out on all that hormonal preparation. Unfortunately the mother doesn't get that head start with the mothering and the baby doesn't get that preparation for life outside the womb. I mentioned before that the baby's more likely to have breathing difficulties, sometimes severe breathing difficulties, more likely to have a low blood sugar, and more likely to have poor temperature control and be just a bit drowsy.

In elective, or scheduled c-section, it's a bit like if you're sleeping in the middle of the night, and someone comes in and wakes you up, and shines a bright light in your face, and pulls off the big clothes, and it's cold, and you're shocked, and the light's too bright, and you just haven't had that preparation that Mother Nature gives us to wake up slowly and gently. That's exactly the same process for the baby.

They naturally have this process, preparation that has them, gently and slowly through labor, through the weeks before labor, getting ready to function very well. To be optimally prepared for life outside the womb. The scheduled c-section baby doesn't get that; it's a stressful experience for the baby.

We know that from looking at the hormones in c-section babies, they have lower levels of stress hormones at birth because they haven't been through labor in birth and haven't gradually had their systems switched on, but they have high stress hormone levels afterwards, and you know, people say for the cesarean baby, this stress comes after birth because they haven't had that preparation.

If the mom hasn't had that hormonal stimulation, we know that her hormones are different during her breastfeeding period (in the case of a c-section). We know that breastfeeding can be more difficult after a c-section as well.

Something to bear in mind if you want to have a c-section and you want to do the best possible way for your baby and really get their help- the other two ways you can stimulate those hormones is:

1. Skin to skin contact with your baby that releases oxytocin that releases beta-endorphin. It calms down your adrenaline. [you'll learn all about this in the next chapter!]
2. Breastfeeding. Three of those hormones: oxytocin, prolactin, beta-endorphin are also released during breastfeeding.

Mother Nature realizes sometimes birth doesn't go according to plan, but this is her backup system, your skin to skin contact with your baby and early and continuous breastfeeding as much as possible. They can really help to familiarize some of that stress for the baby and for the mom as well.

Sarah: That was going to be my follow-up question, … *"How do we get as many benefits and make the best of a c-section?"* and you just answered that beautifully.

Dr. Buckley: One other thing that happens for (scheduled) cesarean babies, because they have not had those weeks of preparation and the mom isn't ready to give birth, the baby hasn't signaled their readiness for life outside the womb.

They usually do that by releasing hormones signaling to the mom's body that they're ready for life outside the womb, which triggers mom's body to begin labor. So the baby might be several weeks away from naturally being ready for labor.

Emergency C-Sections
(C-Sections that start with labor)

Dr. Buckley: The ideal c-section actually lets mom initiate labor with her baby, then if we were really concerned about the well-being of mom or the baby, then we'd proceed with the c-section. We'd do a c-section AFTER mom has gone into labor so mom and baby still get the benefits of hormonal interplay and stimulation during labor.

Research has shown the benefits for babies and the risks of breathing difficulties are not as bad as compared to scheduled c-sections. They aren't quite as good as vaginal births, but somewhere in the middle.

Sarah: Thanks for sharing such really great information Dr. Buckley! How do we wrap this all up? How do we optimize and take advantage of all of these hormones that are working inside of our bodies from the moment we become pregnant?

Dr. Buckley: Know that your body is superbly designed for pregnancy, labor, and birth! You can trust your body and you can trust your baby. You can trust these processes of birth that have developed over millions of years and are perfectly attuned to each other. You can trust birth.

Being better mamas and better care providers are instinctive behaviors. Slow down during your pregnancy. Find a situation where you'll be private, safe and unobserved in labor. Hold your baby skin-to-skin after birth. Follow your instincts, trust Mother Nature's superb design, and you'll reap the rewards in terms of safety, ease, pleasure and health for you and for your baby.

Sarah: Thanks so much Dr. Buckley for helping us to see that hormones are so important to us and our babies. More of Dr.

Buckley's books, webinars, and articles can be found at www.SarahBuckley.com or www.gentlenaturalbirth.com

***

Let's check out this quick overview of hormones; we put them in a chart for you. These are the most important hormones in your pregnancy, birth and while becoming a mama.

6 MAIN HORMONES AT A GLANCE

Oxytocin	Prolactin
• Bonds baby to mom for life! • Causes uterus to contract. • Makes mama chill out. It's called the hormone of calm and connection. • Is released more during labor and birth than any other time. • Turns on the areas we need for mothering. • Causes orgasm during sex. • During sex it bonds the partners together.	• Major hormone of breast milk making. • Hormone of mothering, we release and produce it during pregnancy, it turns on our mothering behaviors. • Reduces stress levels and how susceptible we are to stress.
Beta Endorphin	**Epinephrine Norepinephrine**
Acts as natural painkiller- puts you into altered state of consciousness. I like to call it "gets you in the zone."	Keeps mama alert during labor when those beta-endorphins are kickin' in.
Progesterone	**Estrogen**
• Thickens uterine walls so fertilized egg can implant. • Helps keep a protected and supportive environment for fertilized egg and growing fetus. • Slows down your digestion, so your baby can get all the nutrients out of your food (which is why you might have gas, constipation and heartburn). • Makes us mamas sleepy when we are pregnant. • Teams up with the hormone Relaxin to soften & loosen the cartilage and ligaments so we can grow that baby. • Elevates body temperature during ovulation so the fertilized egg can attach to the uterus. • Progesterone keeps things in line in the placenta and actually prohibits breast milk production while pregnant, so after baby is born and the placenta is delivered, your milk production kicks in.	• Heightens our sense of smell when we're pregnant. It does this by increasing the blood flow to our mucous membranes. • Stimulates the oxytocin system. • It helps our uterus grow. • Prepares breasts for milk production. • It kicks in with your little bambino too and helps their organ development and bone density.

In Short

The way our bodies are designed is IN-freaking-Credible, isn't it? The symphony of hormones masterfully working together in your body right now, are enough to make Mozart green with jealousy.

Just as a symphony tells a story as the music harmonizes, gets louder, softer, super quiet, and gets more intense, so too do our hormones get stronger, softer, quieter and harmonize, moving perfectly together with our baby through labor and birth.

It's easy though to feel overwhelmed by the "what ifs" or "shoulds." It's easy to feel really poorly about ourselves if the birth we so desperately want (for all the benefits that Dr. Buckley explained earlier) doesn't happen, or if we choose a different route.

So here's the deal mama.

You now know A LOT of game changing info here, stuff that 99% of pregnant mamas have no idea about. Even things that many doctors were never taught in school and still don't know. So here's how you use it to have an easier labor and healthier birth: make a plan and set your expectations.

Set your expectations, from the start, based on facts. We will never tell you that getting an epidural makes you a weanie and less of a mom because that is simply not true.

There's no right way to have a baby, but there's a right way for you.

Let's say you have your heart set on moving to San Diego, cause, let's face it, San Diego is awesome. They have awesome weather, beautiful beaches, laid back peeps. It's a great place to live. But you also know that if you move there you'll probably live in a pretty small house (compared to where you live in Lost Springs, Wyoming). You might have to work 2 jobs and will have to deal with traffic and a long commute to work. Is it worth it? You have to decide for yourself. To someone who loves small town life, the trade-off probably isn't worth it. But for someone like yourself who enjoys the ocean, maybe it is.

It's the same type of decision with the epidural and hormones. You and only you can weigh the benefits of the pain relief with the benefits hormones can give you and your baby. Just know that there are tradeoffs that are more likely to happen because of that epidural. It doesn't mean they're guaranteed to happen, but ignoring them or not being educated about them does not serve you or your baby well.

Mama, continue learning and figure out what's right for you and what you're comfortable with. As long as you do that, then you've got nothin' and I mean nothin' to feel bad about 'cause you're doing the work to learn what's best for you and your baby. And that's pretty awesome!

You're only on chapter one and already you've learned how hormones help you become a rock star mom and you FINALLY have an answer as to why you'll now cry during commercials! Plus you're all informed now about how hormones bond you and your baby and help your baby get off to a solid start outside the womb. Aren't you excited? This is just the tip of the iceberg in learning about all these unseen things that will help you and your baby have a healthier birth and start off life on the right foot.

Take Action

1. **Start writing a birth plan.**

   Birth plans are your way of identifying what's important to you. We freaking love them. The reason why we heart them with a passion is that, not only are they incredible communication tools between you, your spouse, your provider, your birth support (doula) and your nurses, they also help you dial down what options you have, and what you want. They're also an easy, effective, way to make sure you're on the same page with your birth peeps. They help you sort through everything you're learning. Putting pen to paper moves you forward. It helps you feel momentum.

You don't have to have it all figured out before you write your birth plan. You just start writing your birth plan to help you figure it out. Just write. Write what you're thinking about. Write something that stuck with you. Write what you don't think you want. Just write. And …

Birth plans set expectations.

The process of writing one, helped Steve and I think through and discuss things that otherwise, we probably wouldn't have chatted about and come to decisions about until we were in the heat of the moment when neither of us could really think clearly.

Half of learning what you DO want is realizing what you don't want.

And in case you're wondering, YES, birth plans are awesome ESPECIALLY if you're having an epidural or a scheduled c-section. There are things you can do during your birth to enhance the bonding, things like skin to skin. We dig into this stuff in chapter three.

Download our Birth Plan Template by putting this link in your browser
http://bit.ly/1ekgPLd

All our downloads are included at the end of this book.

Alright mama, now that we understand the symphony that is happening in your body and the bonding that occurs after birth via hormones, let's now move on to learning about how incredible your baby is. Get ready to freak out at the miracle baby you have inside your womb. Proud parent moments start NOW.

Chapter 2

How to Help Your Baby Take Their First Breath With Less Chance of Complications

with Dr. Lucky Jain MD, Neonatologist, Dad

I was pregnant with my first. And before I ever read one sentence in any pregnancy book or took our birth class, I knew that hearing him scream his little cute head off after birth was going to be a super important milestone in his health. I mean, we all kind of just know that, don't we?

But I never thought at all about *how* he would have to suddenly go from not using his lungs at all in my womb, to successfully using them for every single breath in like 3 seconds flat. I never thought of it as an absolute miracle.

I didn't realize their amazing little bodies had a lot of things to do to make their first breath happen.

I assumed it would just sorta happen, you know?

But after hanging out with Dr. Lucky Jain, I see how silly that is. I mean, when does anything *really* "just happen" totally on its own. I didn't realize there were a ton of things I could do to help my baby take his first breath!

You know, it's almost like going to Hawaii or something … (can you tell I'm writing this in a grey, cold, 15 inches of snow on the ground, Michigan, December?)

You're not going to wake up tomorrow morning on Waikiki Beach by willing it to happen. Things have to happen to make it happen, right? For starters, you have to know Hawaii is an option to go to, then you have to want to go there, then you have to make some money to buy a ticket, you have to buy the ticket, then you actually have to physically get on and then get off the plane and then bask in the amazing smells of paradise as you disembark and get lei'd. Did I seriously just say that?

You get the idea.

Bottom line mama … if there's a place you want to go, there are things you can do to help yourself or a loved one get there.

The same is true for your baby's first breath.

Do you want to help your baby breathe easier after birth (and reduce the chance of respiratory distress, which is one of most common health issues with newborns)? And give them exactly what their little bodies need most to be healthy and thrive?

You can!

There are a few things, that you, as baby's mama, need to know and a few easy action steps you can take to help your baby be as healthy as possible.

This is *incredibly* important information that many birth classes never talk about.

I didn't know there was anything I could do to help my baby take their first breath until I talked with Dr. Jain. He's an amazing man, he's one of the top physicians in the world, he specializes in respiratory disorders in newborn and he's going to teach us HOW our babies take their first breath. I hope you learn as much as I did!

Once you understand *how* your little bundle of cuteness takes their first breath, this book will teach you *how* to help them take their first breath and make it easier for them to get the oxygen they need.

Dr. Lucky Jain is a neonatologist, professor and executive vice chairman for the Department of Pediatrics at Emory at School of Medicine. He also serves as medical director for the Emory Children's Center, he's a chief quality officer, and he's a dad of 2 girls. Dr. Jain also runs the neonatal intensive care unit. That means he specializes in helping babies get healthy and stay healthy. He knows what it takes for babies to thrive.

***

> "It's really critical to know & understand how much the last few weeks (of pregnancy) mean to your baby's health."

> -Dr. Lucky Jain, neonatologist

Sarah: What is the one thing all your experience has taught you about having a healthy baby and that you'd like to share with new moms?

Dr. Jain: There is a lot to be said about believing in Mother Nature and doing birth as naturally as possible. And one particularly important aspect is the fact that pregnancy was meant to be a certain length of time. If moms can remember one thing ... every week of your pregnancy counts ... not one day less and not one week less.

Sarah: Is it true that it's very hard to tell exactly how far along you really are? Due dates are just an educated guess and do not

directly correlate to your baby's accurate biological development?

Dr. Jain: Yes, that is true. Even with the most precise methods available, we still have between a one-week and two week variation in our estimates. That's why I say natural birth is so important, because spontaneous natural labor indicates the baby's biologic maturity and mother's readiness to deliver.

Sarah: You specialize in respiratory disorders in newborns, but before we dive into why every single day counts towards having a healthy baby, you also mentioned there is a unique opportunity in the relationship that physicians and moms can have during birth. And the relationship is really different from any other doctor-patient relationship and can actually improve the health and quality of care moms and babies get. Can you share why you think this relationship is so important for moms to understand?

Dr. Jain: Absolutely! In many other areas of medicine, particularly where critical decisions are made, those decisions are often left to the medical team by the patients (or their families). And we certainly take that responsibility seriously. Whether we are in the ICU or in the general wards, we take ownership of medical decisions and treat patients to the best of our abilities.

Pregnancy and birth is different.

Pregnancy and birth has a very unique opportunity. The level of partnership that exists, or should exist, between an expecting mother and her provider during pregnancy and childbirth is extremely powerful.

I must say, I've practiced medicine now for over 30 years and there is no other area having that level of cooperation, coordination and conversation around important medical decision-making. I wish that we could use this provider-patient model to enhance collaborative care in other areas of medicine.

Sarah: That's a really great point - finding the best provider to be on your birth team, and then using that team to make decisions together. The best decisions are made together. Collaborative care provides the best maternity care because it's focused on getting the best information for each decision for each mom and baby getting care. The best providers know they don't know everything, and are confident in their ability to give better care by working as a team. (Learn what questions to ask and how to find the best doctor or midwife in Birth Book #1)

Ok, let's talk about the baby's transition from living in womb to breathing in the outside world. Can you explain to us what happens between the moment the baby comes out and the moment they take their first breath?

Dr. Jain: I'd be happy to! If you ask a bunch of mothers and obstetricians what the baby's lungs are filled with while they're in utero, the first answer you'll always get is amniotic fluid. They say this because the baby is continuously submerged in a large pool of amniotic fluid.

The first thing to understand is that the fetus is not actually allowing any of the amniotic fluid to get into their lungs. But the fetus is actively making lung fluid [different from amniotic fluid] in very large quantities.

And at birth, this production of lung fluid has to stop. The baby has to begin the task of clearing the fluid out of their lungs so they can create space for breathing in air.

So in the simplest of words, the two major tasks that a transitioning a baby (transitioning from living in the uterus to successfully breathing on their own) must perform are the establishment of spontaneous breathing and circulation into the lungs.

Neither of these tasks occurs in the baby before birth, because the mom's placenta performs all of the functions required by the baby's lungs.

Sarah: That is so fascinating! From the studies I've read and what I'm hearing you say, the baby is pumping that fluid out of their lungs so they can make room for breathing air after birth?

Dr. Jain: Yes, but let me keep going … so early on, the fetus is making a lot of fluid because that serves as the scaffold on which their lungs are actually built.

If you drained that fluid from the fetus's lungs, their lungs would not grow properly. We know that because that's what happens when the amniotic sac membrane ruptures early or babies are not making enough urine.

But after birth, there is a very elaborate mechanism in the lungs that actually clears all that lung fluid out. And it all happens through the absorption of sodium.

There are millions of little molecules in the baby's lung lining that rapidly go to work and absorb sodium. With the sodium absorption, there is also absorption of chloride. The salt movement (from the sodium absorption) draws that lung fluid from inside the lungs and moves it out and into the blood.

We know this, because if for any reason this process doesn't go through properly, the lungs stay wet, and that causes the baby to breathe fast.

In medical terms, we call this condition "transient tachypnea of the newborn," which means for a brief period, the baby is breathing fast.

If the amount of retained fluid in the lungs is a lot, then these babies can have breathing difficulties for up to 3 days after birth. This is a very important mechanism.

Sarah: I've read that another important way that babies can get that lung fluid out is by passing through mom's narrow pelvic passageway, is that true?

Dr. Jain: Not because of any benefit the physical impact through the passage gives. Once upon a time, we used to think that during the passage through the birth canal, the lungs got squeezed, and therefore, helped that lung fluid to get squeezed out. But we now know that is not the case.

Here is what actually happens during active labor in a vaginal birth … the body secretes large amounts of stress hormones, like steroids and catecholamines. Those hormones actually help activate this process we've been talking about, which then clears the sodium and water from the baby's lungs.

So the physical process of passing through the birth canal is a secondary helper to getting that fluid out. Passing through the birth canal is not the primary way the baby's lungs get rid of the fluid.

It's the rigor of labor inducing some level of stress on the baby, which then results in the baby producing stress hormones that aid in clearing out the fluid from the baby's lungs.

Sarah: It's so amazing how this all just sort of happens while you're wiping away the tears after birth. It's incredible how moms' and babies' bodies work together to optimize the babies' birth and health!

Dr. Jain: It absolutely is. It's fascinating!

Sarah: Ok, I'd like to talk about c-sections for a few minutes. Respiratory challenges for babies are fairly common after c-

sections and we know c-section rates are really high in the US (approximately 33% of all women giving birth have a c-section according to the CDC).

Some of us may be medically required to have a c-section. What kinds of things do we need to know, be aware of and what can we actually do, to minimize the chances of our babies having any respiratory challenges?

Dr. Jain: I should start by saying that there are conditions for which cesarean section can be life saving. For example, if there's a large birth defect that would prohibit your baby being delivered vaginally, like a hydrocephalus baby.

But for normal babies who are electively delivered by cesarean birth, it's important to remember that these babies have not had the opportunity to secrete the hormones which would have allowed for smoother transition of extracting out their lung fluid. And so after birth, they generally have larger amounts of fluid in the lungs than their vaginal birth counterparts.

They tend to breathe faster after birth for varying periods of time, and because they breathe fast, they often need oxygen. They often have enough respiratory difficulty to be admitted to the NICUs.

Sarah: Earlier, you said *"every week counts, every day counts"* towards having a healthy baby. You also said to me that there are long-term consequences our babies experience based on the decisions we make during pregnancy and birth. Can you give us an example?

Dr. Jain: Every provider who's been doing this long enough remembers at least one case that in all their life time, will never be forgotten.

And the one I so clearly remember (probably because I narrated the story over and over again in my head), is the case of an army officer who was being deployed to Afghanistan. He wanted to see his baby before he left the country, and so the family in rural Georgia insisted on having their baby delivered at 37 weeks.

That baby ended up developing severe respiratory distress. Subsequently, he was admitted to Children's Healthcare of Atlanta where we had a hard time treating the respiratory failure. The baby survived, but only after being put on artificial lungs.

All of this- just for the joy of "having to see the baby" and being delivered a week or several weeks early. This is the type of *avoidable* disease that we sometimes deal with.

And I think it's really critical to know and understand how much the last few weeks mean to your baby's health.

To help you understand that, I'll use my airplane example ... the last few weeks of pregnancy are akin to a big jumbo jet airplane putting down its landing gear.

If you take away the critical last two or three weeks of pregnancy, it's like taking away two or three critical parts of that jumbo jet's landing gear. Some people somehow think that airplane is supposed to land safely with only half of its landing gear down or sometimes none of its landing gear down. But that plane is not at all in a position to safely hit the runway.

Just like this plane trying to land when it's not ready and not in a safe position to land, so too babies sometimes have a lot more trouble transitioning into the world than we would normally anticipate.

Sarah: So for the baby in that example you gave, what might some of the repercussions be for choosing to bring baby into the world, before the baby was ready?

Dr. Jain: There are some short-term consequences, as you can imagine Sarah, and there are long-term issues that we need to worry about.

The short-term consequences are breathing difficulties requiring intravenous fluid. In the intermediate duration, these babies continue having oxygen needs and therefore cannot be fed by mouth. And if babies don't feed well by mouth in the first week or so, it takes them a very long time to learn how to bottle-feed or breast feed.

Longer-term studies now coming out, particularly from Europe and some from the US, show that these babies often have developmental difficulties. In school age, they have learning disabilities and a bunch of other problems that could have been avoided.

Something else I'll mention Sarah, there are studies I've looked at relating to the microbial colonization of the gut, and one study showed that the bacterial colonization of the gut is different, for up to 70 years, when you're delivering by vaginal birth versus a cesarean birth. Imagine how just one small difference during birth leads to such a striking difference in outcomes for an entire life.

Sarah: What advice or what specific steps would you give to expectant moms as they approach their childbirth?

Dr. Jain: The first thing I'd like to emphasize is that prematurity is a very big problem for us and that the definition of pre-term birth, less than 37 weeks, was actually a man-made definition.

"Pre-term birth" is not a biologic definition.

If a baby is delivered at 38 weeks, don't assume that baby is full maturity. 39 to 40 weeks is when we really start to consider a baby to be fully mature and ready to be born.

And waiting is particularly important if we are going to have an induction or a cesarean birth. The reason it's so important is because in normal spontaneous birth [spontaneous labor and birth is when mom naturally begins labor on her own], you can let Mother Nature take its time, for the most part, and allow the mother to go into spontaneous labor on her own, which indicates full-term gestation for that mother.

[Remember what Dr. Jain taught us above, the baby is the one who actually signaled that they were ready to be born by releasing the hormones which communicated to the mom's body to begin labor]

But if we are going to induce or have an operative delivery via c-section, we better be very sure of dates. That's why early prenatal care or one early prenatal visit for dating of the pregnancy is critical, especially if we get into an area where 30%, 40% or 50% of mothers have some type of intervention. If they don't have good dating of the pregnancy, it becomes a huge problem.

And the final thing I would say is that while obstetricians have a huge role to play in how medical care is provided around the time of birth, mothers need to become educated about the pros and cons, and take a bigger role in how their pregnancies and their childbirth is managed. And after birth, they need to make sure their babies are breastfed and taken care of in the way that will give them the best potential in life.

Sarah: I want to go back to something you just said because I think a lot of people might be surprised that you, as a physician, are strongly encouraging women to take proactive roles in their own healthcare.

There's a perception that doctors are always in charge, they always call the shots and they just sort of show up to make decisions and that's what ends up happening. There's a

perception that I felt as a first time expectant mom (and hundreds of women I've spoken with have also had the same perception), that what I think, feel, say and have concerns about doesn't matter because I'm not a medical professional. It's like our thoughts have no credibility. And if we ask questions and want more understanding of what's happening, there's this perception that we're questioning our doctor or "not trusting" our provider.

But it sounds like what you're saying is that women really need to step up, be proactive, ask tons of questions and make decisions with their provider? Is that what I'm hearing you say?

Dr. Jain: Yes, absolutely! I think hospitals which have the best outcomes – I may not be speaking with a rigorous scientifically done study in my hand, but just from my own experience, I can tell you that the hospitals and practices who have the best birth outcomes have very engaged families and parents throughout the entire pregnancy and birth process.

But is that really any big surprise Sarah?

You see that across the board for anything we could possibly talk about. When you have involved and engaged parents, better outcomes usually happen, right? Whether you look at middle school or early schooling, schools with involved parents tend to have children who do really well.

A baby's birth is particularly an area where if you have an informed mother asking good questions, you can help guide the obstetrician to the right place, so you can avoid an early delivery or avoid a c-section, just because it's most convenient to the provider.

Sarah: Thanks Dr. Jain for all your wisdom, sharing from your 30+ years of experience helping babies get healthy and helping

us learn easy things we can do to help our babies take their first breath!

Dr. Jain: My pleasure Sarah.

In Short

Let's recap what Dr. Jain suggested we do to help our baby take its first breath. But first, let me share something with you which might help you put all these pieces together.

My hubby Steve is a Navy pilot and he now trains other aspiring military pilots in flight school. He tells me about how one of the most important lessons his students have to learn is that they must constantly adjust all the things they're doing, while they're busy flying, with the new information they're getting.

They learn to make constant little adjustments, so they can safely stay on course towards their desired destination, all while minimizing the chances of things happening that they don't want to have happen, in situations (like weather) that they can't completely control.

Sound familiar?

These little, constant adjustments are the secret sauce that make getting to their destination so much easier and safer too.

Pregnancy and childbirth is the same.

We don't have to have *everything* figured out. We don't have to know *exactly* how it's all gonna happen. We don't need to pressure ourselves into believing there's only one way our labor and birth has to happen.

We need to be educated. We need to have a plan. We need to have a provider who wants to help us get to where we want to go.

But most of all ... as we're experiencing pregnancy and labor and birth and becoming a mom, remember that it's good, important and normal to learn as we go! And part of that learning process is making those small, awesome adjustments as we go.

Feel any lighter?

Ohhhh man, when I finally experienced that, I felt a major load off my back.

What did we learn in this chapter?

We can help our baby take his (or her) first breath more easily! Wahoo!

1. Find an awesome provider who will work with you. We have this unbelievable opportunity to partner with our provider as a team in order to make important decisions (which usually results in better decisions that lower risk) and we have no idea this opportunity exists!

The reason the opportunity exists is because birth isn't an emergency situation.

As Dr. Jain points out, we have plenty of time to talk with our provider, read the research evidence (which is actually really easy to do) and decide the best course of action together. There's a big push for "Collaborative Care" (which just means teaming up with your provider and doing this together) in healthcare, because it works. It's improving people's health.

And Dr. Andrew Freeman, director of clinical cardiology at National Jewish Health in Denver, Colorado said *"You're the captain, I'm the navigator. I think having an empowered patient is a blessing."*

When we take advantage of this opportunity, and really go all out in our partnership with our provider, it's like getting in our awesome trainer plane with our instructor. Together, we can make the best little adjustments along our course, so we stay on track towards our target (target being "healthy birth land"). And when we get off track (which we will from time to time), the more we communicate, the faster we get back on track.

2. Allow your labor to happen naturally; on its own.

Remember what Dr. Jain said, "'pre-term birth' isn't a biological definition." Your baby knows when they are "fully developed" and ready to be born, better than *anyone else*. When they're ready to be born, THEY will release a hormone initiating labor. Every baby develops at a different rate. Every woman's body will uniquely begin labor when the time is right. The truth is, nearly every single woman will go into active labor on her own, if given the chance.

Inducing labor or scheduling a c-section before baby is ready for life outside the womb limits their biologic ability to transition into the world in a healthy way (barring an emergency situation of course).

Dr. Jain suggests you allow the timing of your labor to happen as naturally as possible (meaning don't get in the way of it unfolding on its own) so your baby is more fully developed to transition easier during their first breath.

And remember what Dr. Buckley mentioned, even if you need a c-section, talk to your provider, you might be able to allow yourself to go into labor on your own (before the c-section), which would allow for your baby to get some of those important hormones Dr. Jain & Dr. Buckley both talked about.

3. Get an early appointment with your provider to help date your pregnancy.

Dr. Jain also said that in the event an Induction or c-section is medically required, having an accurate dating of the pregnancy is important to help determine how developed the baby is. Ultrasound is often used as a tool to help date a pregnancy. The earlier the ultrasound is done in a pregnancy, the more accurate it is.

You are an amazing life giving woman! Don't forget how powerful and capable you are.

Take Action

1. Remember that birth plan from chapter one? Finish it up and then take it to your next appointment...yes... even if you're only in your first or second trimester. Go through a couple of the items at each of your next appointments and just touch base with your provider to make sure you're on the same page. These are great talking points, especially when they say "Do you have any questions?" and your pregnant brain takes over and draws a blank. Oh yes. I've been there. We all have.

In case you need the link again to our Birth Plan Template. Here it is: http://bit.ly/1ekgPLd

Chapter 3

How Skin to Skin Can Improve Your Baby's Health & Double Your Breastfeeding Success

with Barbara Harper, RN, Midwife, Birth Educator, Founder of Waterbirth International, Mom of 3

Have you ever traveled to another country (or another state) and been knocked upside the head with culture shock? The sights, the tastes, the smells and the language assault every cell in your body. As great as this new place may be, it takes some getting used to. You may experience homesickness and the familiarity of what you left behind.

Imagine your baby being all cozied up inside your body for, basically, 10 months. They've gotten used to your fantastic womb service. Then suddenly they start traveling down and out your body and are now in a foreign land. They need a second to get their bearings.

Skin to skin helps them do that.

Skin to skin care (or kangaroo care) is when a naked, newborn baby (it's okay to wear a diaper) is placed chest down on mommy's bare chest, so mom and baby touch skin to skin. Then, blankets are placed on mama and baby so everyone is warm and snuggly.

This is a "clothing not optional" party. Or I should say, no clothing between you and baby. It's all about the skin mama and you'll understand (and be blown away) why something so simple helps your baby's health. But first, check this out:

> According to the Centers for Disease Control (CDC), only 43% of hospitals do skin to skin for at least 30 minutes within the first hour after birth- and this is for uncomplicated, vaginal births.[i]

This seems like a super low number for something that costs no money, doesn't need any fancy equipment or special training. All it involves is putting your newborn baby onto your chest.

Are we missing something? Or are hospitals?

Barbara Harper is a medical professional … she's a registered nurse, a midwife and travels around the world teaching doctors, midwives, nurses and hospitals about evidence based birth practices.

She's going to teach us *how* your baby's health benefits so much from skin to skin care. She's also going to share the medical research evidence proving *why* your baby's health gets better (it improves your health too). And together, we'll teach you how to ask for it and even give you a script to make it super easy. Let's do it!

***

"The research is clear. One of the best places your baby will transition from womb to world, most successfully, is skin to skin on your chest."

-Barbara Harper, midwife, educator

Sarah: Is there any proven research and evidence showing the benefits of doing skin to skin with your baby right after birth? Or is skin to skin just a "feel good" thing moms talk about doing with their cute newborns?

Barbara: Yes, there is research and evidence. We're going to talk all about skin to skin, also known as kangaroo care, but I need to start with a few stories....

During many of the births I've attended in the last 28 years, there wasn't any other place we'd put the baby other than the mom's chest. So my experience with skin to skin care, before I was even aware there was research and documentation showing all the benefits of skin to skin, is quite vast.

What we saw in those babies who did skin to skin with their mothers immediately after birth was remarkable! Those babies responded vigorously to their new life outside the womb and also to their moms, right away. Some of the babies even lifted up their heads a little bit and looked right into their mother's eyes. They were quiet. They didn't cry. And when they finally did cry, it wasn't for a long, long time.

A lot of those babies with remarkably improved outcomes were born in water, so I naturally thought it had something to do with being born in water. But after attending a lot more births, I realized it didn't matter so much where those babies were born, it mattered that those babies went *immediately* to their mother's chest. The baby getting skin to skin was the reason it mattered.

Let me ask you Sarah, what are the 4 things that happen to your baby in the womb?

Sarah: Uhhhhh …

Barbara: Ok, let me help you out! Here are the 4 things that happen to your baby in the womb:

1.) Your baby gets oxygen
2.) Your baby receives nutrition
3.) They are kept warm
4.) And they stay protected

Your baby is programmed to function in the womb, during pregnancy, with these 4 things constantly happening. They're automatic. And they're critical for your baby's health and development.

Your baby has been neurologically programmed to respond to specific instructions from their brain. They respond, they move, and do everything else exactly how and when their brain tells them to do it. This includes deciding when to be born. We call this the 1st imperative. It's a biological imperative. It's biological programming.

Like we said, when your baby is in the womb, they're nurtured, protected, given nutrition and oxygen. When your baby is born and transfers from the womb to the world, they have to instantly do at least a dozen miracles. Having "transition time" (i.e.- skin to skin) helps them accomplish everything they have to do, because they're not quite one hundred percent independent yet.

Babies are not independent yet, because babies are born with immature brains. Not premature, but immature.

Staying skin to skin gives babies that needed transition and helps them with all of those miracles they have to get done.

If we stayed pregnant for the amount of time it would actually take to grow a baby that was almost fully independent on the basic physiological levels, how long do you think you would have to be pregnant?

Sarah: Based on my friends who have teenagers, I'd say 18 years!

Barbara: Ha! Exactly! Here's the truth … the brain actually matures to the point of intelligent communication, expression of will, self-reliance and things like that at around the 24 to 25 month mark.

With my 2nd baby Samuel, he was very advanced with language at 18 months, had a full vocabulary, and was pointing out street signs, and giving directions … I was like *"Uh oh, I'm in big trouble!"*

So if we were to stay pregnant for around 24 months, we'd actually be delivering an elephant! Babies develop and grow extremely fast in the womb. God has set it up, or evolution has set it up so that the baby's brain is immature for a reason. That reason is because if their brain grew any faster and therefore bigger, it wouldn't fit through our pelvis.

GOOD TO KNOW...

Your baby is growing at lightening speed! According to Mayo Clinic Guide to a Healthy Pregnancy, at week 10 of your pregnancy, your baby's brain will create 250,000 new neurons EVERY MINUTE!!

***

Barbara: The baby is born with an immature brain, so they can actually be born!

But after birth, the baby's brain has to continually develop in order to become intelligent. Where do we want that development, growth and maturation to happen ... what is the best place for that continued development?

We have a choice here.

Is the best place for your baby's development in a little plastic box in the hospital nursery with other babies? Or maybe it's by themselves in a crib?

Neither.

The best place for your baby's development is the exact same environment where your baby was neurologically programmed.

Just like your baby was programmed to develop in the womb, your baby has been neurologically programmed to develop skin to skin on your chest.

What does your baby receive by doing skin to skin?

Barbara: Does your baby receive warmth? Yes, because the mother's skin will automatically regulate the baby's temperature.

Does your baby receive oxygen? Yes, because when your baby first comes skin to skin during delayed cord clamping, [we will talk about that next] your baby gets a boost in oxygen during the placental transfusion of blood.

Does your baby get nutrition? Yes, your baby continues getting all the important nutrients, proteins and oxygen from the umbilical cord during delayed cord clamping (another important reason to do delayed cord clamping) and they can get nutrition from breast milk right away.

We want to leave the umbilical cord intact (we don't want to clamp it or cut it) and put the baby onto your chest, or onto your abdomen.

Does your baby have safety? Yes, they're protected because the mom holds the baby close. Being close to you is the only thing your baby has ever known. Being close to you is everything.

You are their safe place.

So literally as the baby is transitioning from womb to world and has to do all these miracles, by doing skin to skin, we're helping them successfully do that by giving them nutrition, warmth, oxygenation and safety.

So let's just say you can't do skin to skin for some reason (i.e.- an acute medical need, emergency, etc.) and your baby's cord has been cut ... the next best thing you can very easily do is have the baby do skin to skin with the dad. Your baby can still get warmth, protection, and oxygen from the air, but they can't get nutrition from the dad, right?

Your baby is neurologically programmed to find your nipple. But your baby doesn't know your nipple from the father's nipple (yet).

This was pretty funny to see ... you have to prepare fathers that the baby will find a nipple and latch on. When you don't prepare fathers, they get quite the surprise once baby latches on!

I call it bobbing for nipples, the baby looks around and says, *"oh, there's a nipple right there!"* and they go for it.

Sarah: I've seen research that says, during skin to skin, hearing the mama's heartbeat and respiration helps the baby regulate their own breathing. And it's especially helpful if the baby is having some trouble breathing on their own, is that true?

Barbara: Yes, that's exactly right. It's not just hearing your heartbeat, but as I mentioned before, the baby has a neurological program in its brain to function best in this skin to skin environment.

We've seen premature babies and full term babies who are not doing well after birth, almost immediately improve when put in the skin to skin environment.

When I was in nursing school, our normal practice was to clamp and cut the cord right away, then put the baby in a plastic warmer box and take them off to the nursery.

I'd like to give your readers the history on skin to skin and tell you a little story...

Another name for skin to skin care is Kangaroo care. It first became known based on an oral presentation, in 1979, by two doctors from Bogotá, Columbia - Dr. Edgar Rey and Dr. Hector Martinez.[ii]

The two doctors made a visit to a Columbian mountain village, where a grandmother was seen carrying her small grandchild, skin to skin, tucked between her breasts under layers of clothing and wrapped-up to form a pouch. They commented that she was carrying the infant the same way a kangaroo would carry her joey in its pouch. That's how the name Kangaroo Care came about.

So the two physicians decided to see if practicing skin to skin might work in Bogotá, where the daily temperature in their hospital was around 50 degrees. The hospital had no heat, formula wasn't available and a lot of their premature babies died.

I've traveled all over the world, and some places you go, it's interesting that these tiny little hospitals have an infant warmer, but no electricity to actually use them. Go to Ghana, or Kenya, or other places like that and this is where some of the vast research on skin to skin care was done, because skin to skin was all they had.

When these two doctors saw that mothers could be the substitute for the infant warmer, they did a study. Actually, what I'd like to say is that the infant warmer is a very poor substitute for skin to skin!

So anyways, in their 1983 presentation of their study, they reported that kangaroo care provided warmth, nutrition, and bonding to all the premature babies in their care, BUT here's the big one and the most important result they found, the mortality rate dropped by 80%!

These physicians saw an 80% drop in the premature mortality rate, simply from putting the baby back on the mother's chest right after birth.

And if the mother wasn't available, they put the baby on the father, and if the father wasn't available, then they put the baby on grandmothers, nurses or whoever could do it.

We're talking about severely premature babies, like under 1,000 grams, that's like one pound. So that's how the original research was started.

And today, I'm sitting here staring at a huge 283 page bibliography book on kangaroo care. It's one of the most researched and the most interesting presentations for both premature babies and full term babies.

So why wouldn't we want to do something during birth that is research based, evidence based and doesn't cost anything? Why don't we do it in every hospital, birth center and home birth and why doesn't every single provider know this well documented and proven research? Why don't they teach it in med school?

Here's the reason why: because it's not the norm.

The reason why it's not in every place of birth and it's not encouraged by every provider during birth is simply because it's not the norm. Just like water birth isn't in the norm and therefore isn't an option for most women [we are seeing the most cutting edge hospitals install birth tubs and leading providers offer water births]. And just like delayed cord clamping isn't the norm and therefore isn't the standard of care for most births, even though all the best medical research evidence supports and encourages it [we are seeing a few hospitals change their policies making delayed cord clamping the standard of care ... like Vanderbilt University Hospital for example. But these are the exception!]. It's because we've set up medicine and hospital birth in a way to make the protocol run smoothly, not to provide the best evidence based care.

The research is clear … one of the best places your baby will transition, from womb to world, most successfully is skin to skin on your chest.

Skin to skin will regulate your baby's temperature, it'll regulate your baby's heart rate, it'll regulate your baby's breathing and it'll begin creating those neurological pathways in your baby's brain at a much faster rate, than if they're sitting over in the isolette (incubator) that has a warmer.

Sarah, go ahead and ask me any question, 'cause I can feel your brain churning!

Sarah: You can just see all the hamsters spinning in my brain, can't you?!?

Barbara: Yep, I see 'em! They're spinning all around!

Sarah: I was given the advice by an acquaintance to send my baby to the nursery, because she said *"this is your last shot to get any rest."* That actually went against my intuition and it just sort of went against my personal feelings, but I didn't know any of this information that you're sharing with us now. And I was thinking how a lot of us are told that it's best for the baby to be sent away and taken care of by someone else, so we can sleep.

My nurse told me, *"oh yeah, the nurses will just bring the baby to you when they need to eat or need something else."* So I'm just thinking how everything you're sharing doesn't jive with what we might experience.

And what I hear you saying is that it's a completely different mindset. We're confusing who has the highest and most important need.

You're saying *"instead of bringing the baby to me when the baby 'needs something' … the baby needs to stay with me the whole time, because I am ALL they need. They'll get everything they need from me, when they need it. And if my baby has an acute need of some sort, the doctors or nurses can come to our room to give my baby whatever baby might need. Am I hearing you right"*

Barbara: Yes, that's right. Women ask for sleep and that their babies be taken to the nursery because it's been ingrained in our culture and in our thinking that *"oh we've done this hard, hard, work and we have to rest because we're going to have this baby on our own for the next 18 years without any rest, so we better rest up now."*

But that's such a fallacy.

It doesn't make any sense.

Just think about it for a minute.

The reason it's a fallacy is because we're biologically programmed to give our babies the care they need, right when they need it and need us most!

Our hormones that produce the colostrum (which is baby superfood) and breast milk go haywire when our baby is not with us. When our baby is taken away (to the nursery for example), our bodies react as if the baby has died. This is what happens if we don't "receive" the baby and do what we've been biologically programmed to do. It's human physiology. All our bodies know is that our baby isn't there, and they should be.

The power of the hormonal interplay between you and your baby is not to be underestimated.

Your baby has the exact same hormones you do. A "dancing" of hormones between you and your baby is why the mother-child lifelong bond is so strong. Of course you "love" your baby. Of course it "feels good" when you see your cutie pie. But it's more than that, it's chemical. It's human physiology. It's very, very real. When you're flooded with oxytocin, your baby is flooded with oxytocin. When you're flooded with endorphins, your baby is flooded with endorphins.

When you take the baby out of a mom's arms, off her chest and put the baby away from her, her body goes into a hormonal and emotional rollercoaster crisis.

There are some researchers studying the link between mother-baby separation and postpartum depression. They're studying the link, because they see that the rate of postpartum depression in mother's who receive their babies onto the chest are often times lower than when moms don't put their babies directly onto their chest.

Let me define that a little better. You could have your baby on your chest, and then the doctor clamps or cuts the cord and puts the baby over in the warmer. We're not talking about a few seconds on the chest. We're not talking about a few minutes on the chest. We're talking direct, warm, vernix covered, wet infant that has just been born, or out of your womb in a cesarean birth, that goes immediately to your chest.

Skin to skin, ventral surface to ventral surface (meaning your baby's heart right up against your heart) and **you stay that way for a minimum of 2 hours**. I recommend with my homebirth clients, that either mother or father have baby skin to skin for 72 hours.

There are numerous studies that compare the mother's relationship to the baby at 3 months, 6 months, 1 year, 2 years, and even 5 years, when the baby has been taken away or when the baby has had even 1 extra hour of skin to skin and the results will blow you away[iii].

At one year, the baby has more cognitive skills and the mother has more empathy and more relationship with her baby than the mother who did not have that one extra hour of skin to skin. Just one extra hour of skin to skin, and there are even some studies that talk about even twenty minutes of skin to skin.

So here's the thing...

As your baby comes out, we assess them by doing the Apgar test at 1 minute, 3 minutes, 5 minutes. We expect them to do an absolute miracle in that first minute.

DID YOU KNOW...?

Apgar was created in 1952 by Virginia Apgar, an anesthesiologist who needed a way to quickly check out newborns to see how they were affected by the anesthesia used during their birth. The Apgar score looks at 5 areas and rates them on a scale of 0 to 2, this is done 1 to 5 minutes after birth. Then they are added together.[iv] Technically, the highest score possible is a 10 but no baby ever scores a 10, the highest is usually a 9.

Appearance (complexion)
Pulse rate
Grimace (Reflex)
Activity
Respiratory effort

***

Barbara: We want them to cry, which signifies that they're exchanging oxygen. We want them to "pink up" (go from their purplish color to a nice bright pink color), which shows that their capillaries are getting circulation for the first time. We want their ductus arteriosus (inside their heart) to close. We want their lungs to just instantly expand and begin working. We want their liver to start metabolizing fat stores. We want their brain to start functioning. We want them to start sucking on a breast and learning how to suck, suck, swallow and breathe. We want to introduce them to gravity and have them neurologically adjust to all this gravity that they never had prior to the birth. We want to introduce them to the good bacteria, that'll stay in their gut, and a bunch of other stuff...

And we want them to do all that in less than a minute.

The nursery nurses are there, waiting with the warm blanket to receive the baby, then they whisk the baby off and examine the baby to make sure it's ok.

This is seriously crazy.

Would you take the puppy that has just birthed from your beloved dog and wipe it down, give it a bath, suction it, clamp the cord, cut the cord, throw away the placenta and then put that little puppy in a glass box to observe for the first two hours, just to make sure it's ok, then give it back to its mother?

Sarah: After hearing you outline the benefits of skin to skin, it does sound kind of odd that we wouldn't be taught all of this by our providers or in our birth classes. But here's my question ... how does the nursing staff explain why they don't leave the baby with the baby's mom?

Barbara: So much of the "birth thing" is set up to make the baby look like a product. I've heard nursery nurses say *"give me my baby."*

Now they say this with all great meaning and I appreciate nice nurses when the baby is not doing well, but we have to think about what is really happening and have a paradigm shift.

We have to turn our thinking 180 degrees from what is "traditionally" done in most hospital birth environments and look at the best evidence that is proven to improve our baby's health.

We have to look at the 283 page bibliography I'm holding right now in my hands and admit that we've been doing it wrong.

This is not the best way to start a human's life on earth. Our life begins by being "received" between the breasts of the person who created us, just like those two doctors saw the grandmother doing in Bogotá back in 1983. They saw, studied and finally understood that the baby received warmth, oxygenation, nutrition and security from the chest of their mom. And when the baby is skin to skin, everything goes normal.

The best thing a mother can do is to educate herself. Moms need to learn from the YourBabyBooty.com website that you and your husband, Steve educate moms with. Moms need to read about kangaroo care, skin to skin, delayed cord clamping, and waiting for that placenta to come out.

No one can take your baby away from you if the placenta is still attached to the cord and the cord is still attached to the baby.

And so you arm yourself with the knowledge of what is based on proven medical research. And you're going to have to reeducate yourself, because some women will say *"eeewww the baby's dirty, I don't want it touching me."*

Here's what I do … this is the routine I do … I lay down a nice baby blanket on the mother's chest, bring the baby to that nice warm baby blanket, let the baby sit there for three seconds, and then mysteriously remove the blanket. She doesn't even see it happen and this wonderful baby, no hat, no suctioning, no clamping of the cord ...just let them be.

I've seen what happens to the babies and all the benefits to the babies for over 30 years. And you obviously see all the benefits with the excellent education you offer moms on your website.

If I could come up to a pregnant mom or even a mom considering getting pregnant and say *"how would you like at age 2 or 3 to have a child that is bright, alert, engaging, self-regulating, goes to sleep, is a pleasure to be with, is beginning to read and doing all sorts of other cognitive activities, is loving and is a bright, healthy and has never been sick with any childhood illnesses one day in their life?"* If I said that to you, would you sign up for the program that would help make all that happen?

Sarah: Of course, sign me up! But I gotta ask you something Barbara. My sister had a very premature birth. What if the baby isn't doing well?

Barbara: For premature babies, for babies that are sick, even for babies that are on ventilators and can't breathe on their own, or are as small as your hand, the best place for them is skin to skin.

I've even watched pediatricians themselves hold babies skin to skin in hospitals.

It does happen that some babies will be taken away for medical care. When it happens, have as much time skin to skin as possible, even if the baby is in NICU.

We bring the mother in and let her spend as much time as we can skin to skin with her baby.

Did you know many hospital NICUs today are being rebuilt to encourage skin to skin care?

Hospitals are rebuilding their NICUs so there is an isolette and a place for mom to lie down. They're using this really wonderful kind of lawn chair, and you lay back, then the nurse can transfer the baby to you. They also teach you how to pick up your baby from the isolette, put them on your skin and then sit down with your baby.

Even if your baby has IVs, even if your baby is on a ventilator and has other needs like that, rarely is there ever a time skin to skin can't be done.

So the idea is having mom participate fully in skin to skin, so she's still caring for her baby even when her baby has other needs. Research studies show that those babies leave the NICU up to 2 weeks sooner. Those babies gain weight faster and they breast feed faster.

One Mama's Experience With Skin to Skin

"When my husband and I found ourselves in the NICU with our premature son, born at twenty-six weeks gestation, we immediately felt a sense of helplessness, as we had no idea how to help fight for our little one's life. When the staff started explaining skin to skin, or "kangaroo care," and all of its benefits, we were immediately on board. We wanted so badly to do something for him and other than prayer, it sounded like that was one of the best things we could do.

Personally, I was amazed to learn that by holding my son skin to skin, my body could help regulate his body temperature, could help his brain development by getting him into a deep sleep, and that it could help stabilize his breathing. What was probably most remarkable to me was learning that by holding him, my body could sense what antibodies he might need to fight off infection and then my body would produce those antibodies in my breast milk! Wow. I thought, *"Sign me up!"*

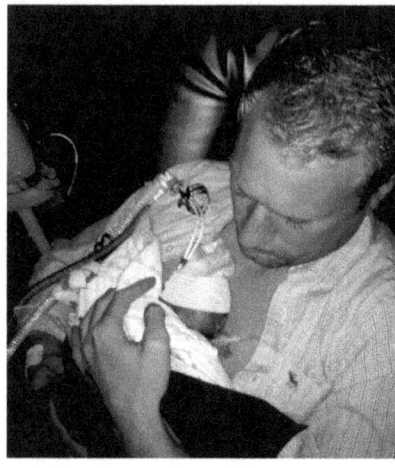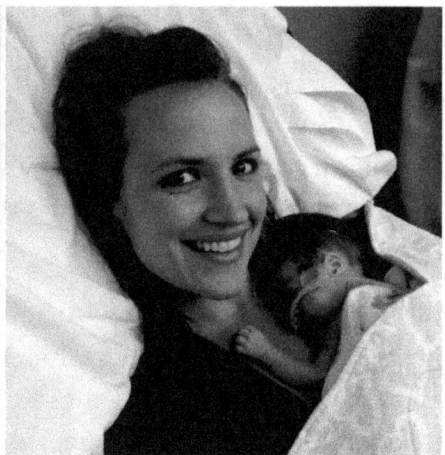

Between my husband and I, we were very fortunate to be able to do skin to skin with our son every day out of the seventy plus days he was in the NICU (except for the first day or two until he was stable enough). It meant me driving one hour each way to the hospital, and James studying for the BAR exam in the lunch room at the hospital, often times in between skin to skin sessions with Brady. It was worth it though, a million times over. Despite being born at twenty-six weeks, we were incredibly blessed that he had no serious long-term issues or disabilities. I can't help believe that the power of skin to skin played a major role in him doing so well.

It's difficult to describe what it felt like, holding my baby to my bare chest for the first time. It was truly incredible and it brings me to tears just thinking about it a year and a half later.

It was so powerful that every time he was close, I could feel my uterus contracting (mostly the first week post delivery), my milk start to let down, my son's heart rate and breathing stabilize. I was quickly starting to experience firsthand the incredible therapeutic benefits of skin to skin for both my son *and* myself.

Everyone in the NICU was impressed with my milk supply, which I attribute to daily skin to skin and a regular pump schedule. The bonding time we shared during skin to skin was priceless, to say the least.

My husband also loved skin to skin and made him feel not only connected to our boy, but helped him feel purpose in a time when we were truly at the mercy of an incredible team of experts.

After having such a positive experience with skin to skin, we both plan on capitalizing on skin to skin with our future baby or babies, regardless of whether they are preemies."
–Katie, James & Brady

***

Sarah: Barbara, what about all the stuff they need to do to baby right after birth?

Barbara: Sarah, let me just say most everything can be delayed for 2 to 3 hours.

Yes, you want to find out how much your baby weighs at birth. But there is no reason that can't wait until later. Optimizing your baby's health is more important, no?

This period is sacrosanct.

When the baby looks into your eyes, and at this place, this distance you see each other for the first time. And when that happens, the baby's pineal gland turns on and starts sending neurotransmitters at 22,000 neurotransmitters a second. They start firing off, and the baby is saying … *"I've arrived, I'm in the right place, I've chosen the right time, I have the right person, I'm* connected. *Hallelujah! Everything is right with the world. The whole entire universe supports my existence and celebrates my being!"*

And when the baby is separated, they go into a chemical and neurological deficit that makes them react sort of like *"is it ok to be here? Is somebody going to rescue me? I don't have enough of this, I don't have enough of that."*

They're just trying to connect to what they're biologically and chemically supposed to be connected to, and their smart little physiology just knows something isn't quite right.

Sarah: Thank you Barbara for this incredible wealth of information. I've been studying birth now for 4 years, I've talked with 100s of doctors, nurses, midwives and other birth professionals and I've never heard all the benefits of skin to skin described like this. I knew skin to skin was super important and beneficial for babies, but I never understood the reason why is because it's the place where they can transition while still getting everything they've been getting inside the womb.

Thank you, thank you, thank you!

***

Another really important benefit of doing skin to skin is amping up your baby's immune system. Dr. Buckley explained this to me in one of our conversations and it's so crucial that I wanted to share it with you, to complete your well rounded education on skin to skin. It's truly amazing how this all works.

Dr. Sarah Buckley: Natural birth is designed to make baby optimally prepared for life outside the womb. Basically you could say it's like waking the baby up.

Your baby goes from a "sleep-like-state" to suddenly having to do all these things their bodies have never done before … your baby has to breathe, to digest, to deal with their own heat-exchange, your baby has to metabolize and excrete, and a lot more.

All those things that your baby's physiologic functions have to do have to happen instantly after birth! So the processes that happen during labor and birth are designed to wake the baby up, so they can function independently.

What happens for the baby during labor and birth actually *optimizes* the baby's physiology for good and probably for their entire life.

One example of how the baby's physiology is optimized during normal birth centers around the baby's gut flora. There is a lot of interest in how humans colonize their gut in recent years.

The gut flora that the baby inherits naturally from the mother, during birth, is a very important immunological resource for the baby. That gut flora provides the backbone for the baby's immune system for their entire life.

[How healthy our bodies remain as adults] has something to do with the immunological process that happens when the baby gets the mother's gut flora during labor and birth.

Sarah: So this gut flora exchange happens during labor AND birth?

Dr. Buckley: We're beginning to understand more and more about that. The classical thing we've seen is that when baby is still in the womb, they're encased in the membrane with amniotic fluid inside. The baby is generally sterile inside the womb; there are no germs inside.

But now we're beginning to understand there actually is some bacterial activity at that stage, particularly once the membrane's rupture, once the water breaks. Then there's a conduit. There's a channel from the mother's vagina that the healthy bacteria travel along to reach the baby.

So after your water breaks during labor, your baby begins getting colonized by the good bacteria. Particularly during birth and postpartum, the baby's colonized by the bacteria that are in the mother's vagina. The baby swallows the bacteria; it travels down and colonizes their gut ... that's how the initial colonization of the baby happens.

Your baby is part of your environment, so the baby is being exposed to the environment they're ultimately going to have to live in. All this good bacteria they get in their gut is what helps them fight off all the bad bacteria they encounter in the real world.

So your baby's gut gets coated with all the good stuff that will fight off the bad stuff. That's a good thing!

Then the baby is born and they have no bacteria on their skin (because the amniotic sac was sterile for the most part), so doing skin-to-skin immediately with mom helps the baby's skin get colonized by the mother's skin flora. Skin-to-skin with mom is so important for babies!

If it's not possible with mom, then dad is second best. But you want someone from the baby's own home environment, because bacteria from the home environment are the bacteria your baby will have to first fight off once they're in your house.

Doing this will optimize your baby's bacteriological environment or your baby's "microbiology" as we call it. It helps your baby stay healthy throughout their entire life.

Keep an eye on this topic. It's really something we're beginning to understand a lot more about, and seeing the long-term importance of having a healthy gut flora for lifelong health and well being.

Sarah: I've talked to a lot of doctors and I've never heard about this with skin-to-skin. I've never heard how skin-to-skin helps colonize our baby with healthy bacteria, which ultimately helps them be self-sufficient at fighting off bad bacteria throughout their lives! It's fascinating.

Dr. Buckley: There was one interesting study done in 1970, and they looked at babies within 1 week of each other in England and Wales. They followed these children up as they got older, and found a correlation between babies that went to the nursery (a lot of babies went to the nursery in 1970) and asthma and allergies at age thirty.

They suspect that maybe the babies didn't get those extra big doses of the mother's bacterial flora by being skin-to-skin or being in the mother's close vicinity. The baby has to be colonized with something, and if it's not the mother's healthy flora, it will be someone else's flora.

In fact, people that handle the baby can pass along bacteria on to the baby, but that's not normal for the baby or healthy for the baby. It's another really good argument for not passing your baby around after birth ... the baby is designed to be skin-to-skin with the mom. The baby needs to be on her body to be colonized in the early days and weeks with the flora that will help them most.

DID YOU KNOW...?

Gut Flora is bacteria that lives in your gut. Experts estimate that as many as 100 trillion bacteria can live there! Gut flora impacts health in many different ways. Here are a few things gut flora does:[v]

1. Extracts energy from food.
2. Boosts the immune system, by fighting the bacteria that causes sickness.
3. Protects against the growth of pathogens, which is a fancy word for disease causers.
4. Produces vitamin k, which builds strong bones, helps blood to clot, prevents heart disease and more.

If you've had a c-section and you're wondering how in the world your baby is going to get the gut flora party started, don't fear, we have 4 ideas for you:

1.   **Skin-to-Skin**- We talk about this in great detail in chapter 4, just know that if you have a c-section, you can still do skin to skin and we show you exactly how.

2.   **Breastfeed**- breast milk is the most complete form of nutrition for babies. When we nurse, we're passing powerful antibodies to our baby. In fact, if someone sneezes in a room while mama is nursing, her body automatically kicks up its production of important antibodies to fight sickness and passes them along to baby in the breast milk. Isn't that cool?

3.   **Mimic the transfer of gut flora from mama to baby.** One couple, whose baby was born via c-section, took a *sterile* cotton swab and transferred some of mama's vaginal secretions to the skin of their baby (you can read about it in this New York Times Article)[vi]. This is not widely done, but what a great idea!

4.   **Start your infant on probiotics.**[vii] Probiotics are essentially "good bacteria", microorganisms that fight disease, sickness & help with digestion. One way you (and your baby) can get these "good bacteria" is by taking probiotic supplements. There are many types and brands. Go to your local experts, your health food store and ask them for recommendations.

***

Sarah: Is gut flora kind of like probiotics? I know those are becoming more popular for women and children to take.

Dr. Buckley: Yes. That's exactly right.

If we have a healthy gut flora then we have healthy digestion and a healthy immune system. We also just learned recently that the gut flora actually helps make some of our brain's hormones. Like serotonin for example, it's the happiness hormone. So I guess when people say, *"your happiness lives in your gut"* ... that's true!

And I think the interest in probiotics is really good, because the mother has to have a healthy gut flora to pass it on to her baby, and many of us don't. We, as a society, probably got the worst gut flora we've ever had in human history for various reasons (one being the widespread use of antibiotics, because it wipes out the good bacteria).

Probiotics and even fermented foods are a really great idea for pregnant moms, because moms can increase their gut flora and pass a healthy gut flora along to their babies.

Sarah: Thanks for helping us understand why it's important for our babies to get our good bacteria! As a parent of two kiddos, I see everyday why it's important to establish that good gut flora early on. Having sick kiddos is heart wrenching.

Supporting Evidence

Barbara mentioned the research done at 1, 3, 5 years after birth that looked at mother and baby interaction. There's this study [viii]published in 2009 by K. Bystrova, in St. Petersburg, Russia which looked at 176 mama-baby pairs. These pairs were split into four groups. In the first group, babies did skin to skin with their mamas after birth and then "roomed in" with them in the hospital. In the second group, the babies were dressed. Their mamas held them and they roomed in with them. In the third group, the babies were kept in the nursery after birth and the entire time their mama was in the hospital. In the fourth group, the babies were kept in the nursery after birth but roomed in with their mamas during their hospital stay.

The results of this study showed that one year later, the skin to skin contact or early suckling or both when compared to separation, positively affected the infants' sensitivity to their mama. It also positively affected their self-regulation and how they reciprocated towards their mama.

This is an entire year later!

So the interaction between mom and baby is positively affected, not just for the time during the actual skin to skin, but one year later as well. That's a huge return on only a few hours investment, isn't it?

Remember how Barbara talked about babies being "biologically programmed" and how skin to skin also has significant positive effects on moms' brains?

The study[ix] Barbara was talking about, says "According to mammalian neuroscience, the intimate contact inherent in this place (habitat) evokes neurobehaviors ensuring fulfillment of basic biological needs. This time may represent a psychophysiologically 'sensitive period' for programming future physiology and behavior."

That basically explains why moms and babies create such a strong lifelong bond.

That's why we sometimes have that "I want my mommy" feeling during challenging times (even as adults). Moms were the first place we ever felt safety and had all our biological needs met for survival. Moms made our challenges and problems go away (i.e.- hunger instantly disappeared with the closeness of her warm boob).

So our brains were hard wired to associate mom with safety, comfort, relief, rest, food, and problem solver extraordinaire. Our brains were programmed to want more of mom.

And mom's brain became hard wired and programmed to want more of baby. The more she met baby's needs, the better she felt (more oxytocin was flowing through her body) – she felt more needed, wanted, validated and accepted for who she was.

Skin to skin improves the bonding ("biological programming") between baby and mom because it increases the brain's release of the exact hormones that cause the bonding.

As Dr. Buckley quoted in chapter one "it's the beginning of a great love affair…"

Researchers looked at 34 randomized studies with 2,177 mamas who had just given birth[x]. The results showed that mamas who did skin to skin after birth had babies who cried less, and actually interacted more with their mama (we usually don't think about newborns interacting at all, so that's really neat!) than those babies who had "usual hospital care." And the babies who had early skin to skin were more likely to breastfeed in the first one to four months of baby's life and tended to breastfeed longer.

In this study published in the Journal of the American Academy of Pediatrics[xi], researchers came to the conclusion that skin to skin influenced "motor system modulation" in newborns. In plain English, this means that skin to skin influences how your baby adjusts its motor system (responsible for movement).

The World Health Organization (WHO) recommends that all newborns, no matter when, where, how, how early, how late they were born, do skin to skin. They wrote a super sweet pamphlet that goes into detail the research and how to do skin to skin effectively. It's on their website.

Mamas who do skin to skin say they are less stressed when doing skin to skin, like Katie shared above, she felt a lot more relaxed and so did her son, Brady. Mamas say that they have more confidence, self-esteem and are more fulfilled, according to a book published by the Neonatal Network.[xii] You will see this theme again when you read the "In Short" section next, as I share my personal experience.

In Short

Skin to Skin at a Glance

Benefits for Mama	Benefits for Baby	Risks for Mama & Baby
Easier & Increased breastfeeding success	Heart rate, temp & breathing more stable	None
Less anxiety at 3rd day after birth	Effective sucking at first breastfeeding session	
Mamas feel more confident	Less crying	
Improves bonding	Improves bonding	
Less breast engorgement and pain at 3rd day	Baby colonizes gut with good bacteria from mom (or dad) which helps immune system	
Increases oxytocin production which turns on mothering.	Increase in blood sugar (a good thing)	
Mama-baby bonding & interaction is positively affected for years to come.	Helps baby transition to life outside the womb.	

After interviewing Barbara Harper about skin to skin, we talked for several minutes on the phone and I shared something with her that I didn't record. Something that still tears me up into little bits when I think about it, something that will always be present in my mind and tinged with regret. And I'd like to share it with you now in hopes that you can avoid this from happening to you.

When I gave birth to our first baby, our son, (who is now 4 years old), I didn't know a fraction of what I know now about pregnancy, birth, skin to skin, or how my body works with my baby to bond and be close. After a relatively short, 8-hour labor, and what I would call a routine, uneventful birth (the kind where everything goes well, without any hitches), I met my baby. I was floored by that moment. I snuggled with him for a few minutes before they whisked him away to measure, weigh, and do all those administrative things could have absolutely waited.

Then I noticed that they didn't bring him back.

The nurses said he had some respiratory things going on (I didn't understand what that meant) and that they needed to take him into the nursery to keep an eye on him.

Knowing what I know now, I would have insisted on skin to skin first, to give him time and help transitioning to a normal breathing pattern, to keep him warm on my chest, to give him all the time his little body needed to experience this miracle of living outside my womb. Knowing what I know now, I am convinced that given more time with skin to skin, that he would have been just fine. Knowing what I know now, when they told me they were taking him, I would have said *"no, my baby stays with me. You guys monitor him here while he's on my chest"* or as an absolute last resort, I would have followed him there and held him skin to skin in that nursery.

Instead, after repeatedly asking the nurse where he was, and then having my friend literally go down the hall, track the nurse down and say *"where is this baby, it's been 4 hours?"*, then schlepping down to the nursery in my bathrobe, and seeing him lying there in an isolette, all by himself...even though I didn't know what I know now, my heart broke into a million pieces thinking of how alone he must have felt, wondering where his mommy and daddy were. I'm tearing up now, 4 years later just thinking about it.

I'm tearing up because I now understand it wasn't just my emotions tugging on me. His little body, mind and spirit needed me. All of me. And he needed me more than he needed a warmer in the nursery and most definitely more than the nurses needed a convenient place to "watch him." No question.

It turns out he was just fine, he needed a little bit of time to transition to life outside the womb. I often wonder how that impacted him and how it impacts him today.

Now some people say (with stuff like this), *"Awww, he's fine, look at him now running around everywhere..."*

I understand what they mean. But sometimes I think people say that just to make me feel better. Now, I'm not going to sit here and think about this and dwell on it and heap burning hot coals on myself. But, remember those "course adjustments" we talked about in the last chapter? This is a perfect example of adjustments. With our next baby, we did skin to skin continuously for about 72 hours. Because we knew the incredible benefits.

Steve did skin to skin with Emersyn during that time as well. Actually we have a video where Emersyn and her big brother meet for the first time. Steve was doing skin to skin with her at the time, and you would SWEAR watching that video that he was the one who gave birth to her. Haha. Serious.

Back to our firstborn, Jackson: we'll never really know how that time apart impacted our son, but I do know that it impacts me.

I had a strong, strong urge to hold my baby those 4 hours while he was being "observed", my hormones were doing their job and opening up this mothering side of myself that didn't previously exist. It didn't feel right to me not to be holding my baby. And my breasts were all *"well baby is gone, so we're done."* Breastfeeding wasn't super easy to get going. We definitely had our moments of struggle.

Looking back on the situation and based on the best medical research evidence available - there was no reason for him to be put in the nursery for observation.

He was put in the nursery because that was the hospital norm. It was just what they were used to doing. Standard hospital procedures trumped proven medical evidence. They didn't know the proven medical evidence. How does this happen?

Those hours he was in the nursery, I could have been doing skin to skin with him while they monitored him more closely. Because I understand that the hospital needs to take precautions and they only have so many nurses available. So we're not saying that it has to be one or the other. It could be the best of both! Me in the nursery doing skin to skin they he was monitored. Jackson's breathing would have regulated faster and we would have optimized the oxytocin surge, the bonding and all the other benefits we learned about above. That is my true regret.

Here's the hope: knowledge is power. You and I now know the power of hormones and skin to skin.

You now know that it's not just feel good, mamby-pamby stuff we're talking about. This is real. It's how human physiology works and more importantly, it's how your baby's physiology will thrive. And it's backed up by tons of medical evidence and research.

There are no risks of doing skin to skin, only lots of benefits. It costs you nothing. It costs the hospital nothing. And something Dr. Buckley mentioned above- you help your baby get their gut flora going too.

Some hospitals proactively offer mother-baby friendly care and promote skin to skin care. But those hospitals are rare and unfortunately, many hospitals do not. Many of you will have the experience where the hospital makes it difficult, in some way, for you to give your baby skin to skin care. Maybe they say that they want to "*observe your baby in the nursery because their breathing has some abnormalities.*" Maybe the nurse or doctor actually says aggressively, "*that's not how we do it here.*" Maybe someone well intentioned says "*we need to clean your baby first.*"

The reasons or excuses don't really matter. What matters is that you Mama, yes YOU, the
"*I'm a first timer, and I don't know anything about any of this*"
mama, YOU speak up and say:

> "*According to the best medical research and evidence, skin to skin helps babies regulate their breathing, body temperature and a bunch of other health benefits. I'd like to do that for a couple hours first before anything else is done and then re-evalute, how about that? Here is the evidence if you'd like to read it.*[xiii]"

If skin to skin is something you want, YOU need to be your baby's strongest advocate (and sometimes politely, aggressive advocate)!

There is a big gap between what the best medical evidence based care is (known by leading maternity care providers and some educators) and the care most of us moms actually get.

The reality is many doctors and most nurses do not know this evidence exists. I know it's hard to believe that you'd go through all those years of med school or nursing school without learning this research evidence, but it's true. They will not be able to rattle off all of these proven benefits your baby gets. They won't know why these benefits actually happen. If they know about skin to skin, they'll likely only be able to say *"I've heard it's good for the baby."* They just can't give you the best evidence based care when they don't even know what it is. That's why it's important for us to speak up!

As I finished telling Barbara this story, I started crying. I didn't realize the impact it had on me, now, four years later. I didn't realize how self-doubt and not listening to my gut instincts really affected my confidence as a mom. Barbara was so kind and loving in her response, encouraging me not to look back, but to look forward and help other mamas avoid this same regret.

Mama, learn from my regret and most importantly check out what the research evidence says for yourself. Listen to your gut instincts and expect that you won't get evidence based care. That way you'll be prepared to insist on getting it.

Politely insist on skin to skin, even if it means following the nurse to the nursery and doing it there, so they can observe your little one. The confidence you'll gain as a mom, not to mention the amazing bonding that you'll get with your baby will serve you well for life.

Take Action

How to get skin to skin
after your baby's birth:

Use this link to download & print these scripts (the
summary of evidence is in here too).
http://bit.ly/1bEc509

1. **Ask for it**. Don't wait until you're at the hospital, in labor,
   or baby is coming out to discuss this with your provider.
   Talk to your provider at your prenatal appointment. Have
   you ever heard the phrase "you don't get what you don't
   ask for"... it's true! Here are some suggestions on what to
   say to you provider:

   **"Do you promote and encourage skin to skin immediately
   after baby is born?"**

   If they say anything other than *"yes, we encourage skin to
   skin and do everything we can to help all our moms have
   it"* ... then you ask:

   **"Are you familiar with the latest research evidence that
   supports it?"**

   If they say "yes", then you say:

   **"So you're familiar with Dr. Edgar Rey and Dr. Hector
   Martinez who discovered the incredible benefits of
   Kangaroo Care (skin to skin) in Bogota Columbia and saw
   their mortality rate drop 80%"** –then you print out the
   summary of evidence from the link above and hand it to
   them.

   Then you say:

"I want to be crystal clear with you now, so there is no confusion during my birth ... I want skin to skin with my baby. My husband and I would love to have increased success in breastfeeding, less anxiety, and better bonding. We'd love for our baby to have an easier time transitioning outside the womb, have easier time with respiratory adjustments, regulation of body temperature and getting their heart rate into a settled rhythm just like the best research and evidence shows. We would love to spend the first two hours getting to know each other and would like for you guys to wait to measure, weigh and assess baby until after we're done, or do it while baby is on me. I need to know you're committed to making this happen for us, even if you're not on duty, are you and your co-workers committed to helping us get skin to skin immediately after birth?

Ok Great! How will you help us make that happen?"

If they sound wishy-washy in any way, and don't say *"yes"* out loud and don't give you a clear commitment that they'll work hard to make sure you get skin to skin (moms have told us they've heard doctors say things like: *"we have protocol we have to follow"* or *"our nurses do what the hospital protocol wants them to do"* or *"I can't help you if I'm not there"* or *"it doesn't really matter that much"*), then you say:

"I'm sure that you practice based on medical research evidence, right? I'm sure the nurses, and the hospital would love for us to walk away from our birth experience satisfied and recommending you and the hospital to all of our friends and family. Nothing would make us happier than being able to spend this important "golden hour" after birth with just our immediate family. That's one of

the reasons we hired you, because we trust that you would work with us to ensure that our birth is accomplished with evidence based practices. I need to know you are committed to making this happen for us, even if you're not on duty, are you committed to helping us get skin to skin?

Ok Great! How will you help us make that happen?"

If they still object, you should think about finding a new provider. If they're this wishy- washy when you're asking for evidence based care while sitting in an appointment, what will they be like when things are moving and grooving during labor and birth?

***

Find someone who supports you, encourages you, believes in you and will give you the care you want. And need. These kinds of doctors are out there! Here's another plug for reading Birth Book #1, where you'll meet a few of these kinds of doctors and we show you how to find them.

If this isn't possible, then schedule a visit with the hospital administrative staff, usually they have a patient relations department. You are a customer paying the hospital, on average, $18,000 for your birth. When you pay $18,000 for anything, don't you make sure you get what you're paying for? You have leverage mama, don't be afraid to use it.

Go over the evidence (start at the top of this page with the scripts), provide them with copies of the research that you printed out. Help educate them about this research.

Here's the thing ... there isn't anything to object to here (except your persistence might cause them to have to break their routine). You're actually helping them practice and provide the best evidence based care. Making the nurses wait to measure, weigh and bathe your baby is NOTHING, compared to the lasting benefits you and baby will receive. You can always offer to weigh, measure and bathe baby yourself if it's that inconvenient for them.

2. **Write it in your birth plan.** Write down that you would like baby placed on your chest immediately after birth to do skin to skin for a minimum of one hour and that baby can be assessed right there on your chest. 'Cause we now know that an incubator has nothing on your chesty-festy mama.

    If you are overwhelmed with the whole idea of a birth plan, here's the link again to our template. http://bit.ly/1ekgPLd

***

Woo mama! You're rockin' and rollin!

Since we've talked about all the benefits of skin to skin and how they are off the hook at facilitating some major miracles for our little ones (and us too), let's dive into skin to skin for c-sections and figure out how that works together.

Chapter 4

How to Get Skin to Skin With Your Baby During a C-Section

with Mavis Schorn, CNM, PhD, Associate Professor of Nursing, Mom

You've read about all the incredible, fantastic benefits for baby (and you) and you really want to do skin to skin. You want in on all these amazing miracles going on. But what if you are having a c-section?

Think about all your friends who had c-sections who never mentioned any of this skin to skin fabulousness. Don't worry mama. You don't have to be left out of this skin to skin party.

This chapter will help you get skin to skin even if you're medically required to have a c-section. Yippeee!

According to the Centers for Disease Control (CDC), only 32% of mamas do skin to skin after an uncomplicated c-section delivery within 2 hours. That is a huge bummer and just doesn't have to be. It doesn't mean that you can't have skin to skin with your baby, it just means you have to be super intentional about getting it.

The standard of care (i.e. what's usually done) for c-sections in the United States is that baby is delivered in the operating room, and then taken to a baby warmer where baby is checked out, weighed, assessed and all wrapped up. Then daddy or birth support walks over, sees and holds baby and brings baby to the mama who gets to see her sweet bundle of joy just for a moment. Then baby is taken away to the nursery where they observe her until the mama is finished with surgery and goes to the recovery room. On average, the separation is 1 to 2 hours.

As you've learned, this first hour of life (the golden hour) is the most important time for mama and baby to be together. The health benefits for baby and mom are medically proven.

Hospitals are starting to listen to their expecting mom patients (also known as customers). They are starting to realize that the way things have "always been done" doesn't mean they can't change, get better and improve for the sake of those mamas and babies.

Moms want better care. Moms are asking more questions. Moms are expecting their doctors and hospitals to actually give their babies care based on proven medical research, and not care based on "normal protocol" which has no medical evidence to back it up and in many cases actually goes against the evidence. We like to call this the "old school" approach.

There are several research studies showing that skin to skin within an hour after a c-section is possible and has no adverse effects. Since one of the pitfalls of a c-section, according to research[xiv], is lack of early breastfeeding, which can lead to breastfeeding challenges from that point on, this is incredible news!

If it's possible for skin to skin to happen after a c-section, the obvious question begging to be answered ... "well then why doesn't it happen in more hospitals?"

One of the biggest reasons hospitals say they can't (or won't) do skin to skin, is because babies born via c-section have a greater possibility of hypothermia. If you've been in an operating room before, you'll probably remember how cold they keep the temp.

Mamas may have a lower body temperature, and so might the baby because of the medications they were exposed to while still in mama's womb. But research[xv] shows that babies who do skin to skin 30 to 50 minutes after birth are not at risk for hypothermia.

I mean, how could they be, all snuggly up with their mama, compared to those babies who hang out in the warmer? And even if mama's body temp is lagging, babies can still do skin to skin with dad or another family member.

The second reason that more c-section babies don't do skin to skin after a c-section is simply because *"it's not the way they do things"* in the operating room. The culture of the operating room is one of tradition and protocol.

Surgeons, nurses and anesthesiologists thrive on established ways of doing things, and for good reason. During surgery, it's important to have a rhythm and method, keeping everyone on the same page. But the best hospitals continuously improve. The best doctors, midwives and nurses ALWAYS find ways to improve the care they provide for the wellbeing and safety of their patients. So guess what ...

Hospitals need to be challenged to change the status quo.

(Doctors and nurses have told me over and over how frustrated they are because their hospitals won't wake-up out of their bureaucratic slow-moving slumber to offer the best evidence based maternity care to women and babies. They get frustrated because sometimes their hands are tied.) Especially when the improvements improve lives and the health of patients. As we'll see later, doing skin to skin doesn't affect the workings of the OR. We're not introducing a new untested surgical procedure here, we're simply changing outdated protocol that actually prevents baby and mama from having optimal health.

I spoke with Mavis Schorn, a mom and Certified Nurse Midwife who has attended over 2,000 births, and is Associate Professor at the Vanderbilt University School of Nursing- I asked her *"How can we have the best bonding with baby with a c-section?"* She shared how and what Vanderbilt is doing to make things more "family friendly." In case you didn't know, Vanderbilt is a big time leader in women's healthcare. They set the bar and lead the way.

As Mavis will share in a story she tells, one good question to your provider could totally change your birth experience AND the birth experience for other mamas too. Check this out.

***

"Your birth makes up a very small number of your life experiences.

And those experiences are precious...so why not shape each one?"

-Mavis Schorn, CNM, PhD

Sarah: People may be thinking *"All right, she's a midwife. She's a mom. She's caught 2,000 babies. Why are we talking about c-sections with a midwife?"* The reason is because Vanderbilt University is a cutting edge and progressive healthcare provider. They're always trying to improve labor and birth for moms. They're discovering a new way of thinking about c-sections and how to make them more family-friendly. So what does that even mean and what would that look like for moms?

Mavis Schorn: Sure, let me tell you the story about how it came to be. An article came out about a doctor who was really trying to improve how a mom experienced her c-section. A couple of us were talking about it, so I sent the article over to our physician who oversees "labor and delivery care" and said *"Hey, check this out. What do you think about this?"* And he was like, *"Sure. I'm on-board. Let's do it!"*

Right after that, we had a woman come in who needed a cesarean because of some circumstances surrounding her birth, and she had a doula with her, and the doula used the phrase *"natural cesarean"* or *"family-centered cesarean,"* I don't remember which one exactly.

But the physician that I sent the article to happened to be the attending surgeon that day. And the anesthesiologist that day was a very open-minded anesthesiologist, and she was like, *"Hey, yeah, why can't we do this?"*

So we had the nurses onboard, the surgeon onboard, the anesthesiologist onboard, the doula onboard and we also got the pediatric team onboard.

We all worked together, with this woman, to make her cesarean the best possible family-centered experience she could have.

We knew we needed to ask some questions about how we needed to do things, so we could improve her experience.

When you think about a mother who, at the very beginning, walks into the operating room, we started asking questions like ... *"What could we do to make even just walking in the room, a far better experience for her? Could we dim the lights? Could we have music playing?"*

And we said ... *"Of course we can. Why not?"*

So we got everybody onboard.

Then we asked questions like … *"Can the EKG attachments we normally attach to her chest be put on a in such a way that they'll still allow for her baby to be placed right on her chest for skin to skin? Can we make sure her arms are free to move around, so she can hold her baby after the birth?"*

And we said … *"Yep, we can do that too!"*

We kept asking questions and tried to come up with answers that would help our moms have the best c-section experience possible.

Here's another example …

Whether a baby is being born vaginally or by cesarean, when the baby's head is out, the baby still receives oxygen through the cord. So even with the cesarean, when the baby's head is out, we've started lowering the drape so mom can look down and see her baby (she still can't see the incision).

And so the mom sees her baby as her baby is being born. Then, the surgeon does something that we call "walking the baby out." The surgeon very slowly lets the uterus actually express the baby, by gently guiding one shoulder, then the other shoulder, then all the way out. So the mother gets to experience and feel something as close to a normal birth as possible, even though a cesarean is medically required.

Then we leave the cord alone and do delayed clamping if the baby is doing well.

As I mentioned, the surgeon is helping the baby birth slowly, so as the head comes out slowly, the mom can look into her baby's eyes right away and babies often cry with just their head out. As they cry and get that oxygen into their blood, their color turns pink, and you can see them transition even before they're all the way out.

There's no urgency to this.

Right when the baby comes out, we delay the cord clamping for a bit, then the baby goes right on top of mom for skin to skin. Like a vaginal birth, we might lightly dry the baby while they're resting on top of mom. The baby can smell and hear her mom.

This is often done in Europe, you dry the baby right there on top of the mom, so mom and husband can see their baby transition, just like a vaginal birth. Then the drape goes back up to maintain sterility, and the surgeon can finish the surgery.

But here's a major benefit ...

The mom is now focused on the baby.

Not the surgery.

When the baby is ready to nurse, the baby can nurse. Mom might need a little help while she's lying flat for the surgery, but babies start rooting naturally right away. They start looking for mom right after they're out.

Do you get the idea? Hopefully I've painted a picture to help you see there are quite a few things we can easily do to help moms have the best cesarean experience possible.

The main point is this Sarah ... a baby is being born here. All of us need to stay focused on your baby and on you. We don't want to be focused on the surgery.

Sarah: That's a really great point! I've talked with many physicians who agree with everything you've said and have told me *"Sarah, we've become way too focused on the wrong thing. The surgery is nothing more than a tool aiding in the birth. Birth is the event. It's important we switch our focus back to the birth."* And I've also talked with many women who get frustrated and think *"oh yeah, my hospital won't go for that. I*

probably won't have an open-minded physician, anesthesiologist or nurse."

But the message you're sending is this ... *"You'll never get what you don't ask for. Stay focused on meeting your baby and ask questions!"*

You and your baby are worth asking for mama! What if that woman who came to Vanderbilt never mentioned "family-centered c-section" in passing? A ten second question completely changed her entire experience. And she'll have it with her forever!

My husband, Steve, is known for asking for discounts for everything. I mean he'll be in Lowe's buying a refrigerator, and he's like, *"Is this the best price you can give me?"* While I'm cowering in the corner afraid they'll laugh us out of the store, he's getting $100 bucks off a fridge that's not on sale.

So the message is "why not ask?" If they say no, you haven't hurt anything, but if they say yes, that could be a really huge moment for you. And your hospital needs to know the best hospitals in the country are improving c-sections for women. They might not be aware it's possible, because they, like many hospitals, are often just stuck in their way.

Can women ask their care providers questions like this? Is there a best way to go about it?

Mavis: First off, you make great points! This whole discussion really needs to happen before labor and birth. This is something women need to feel comfortable talking about with their provider, whoever that is.

There are things we can't control about our birth, but what if asking a simple question could change the entire course of your birth?

119

Asking some *"what if this"* and *"what if that"* questions are absolutely acceptable and expected. Women can ask us questions.

If your questions are received by your provider in a hostile way or you're shut down, that's not right. There are exceptional caregivers, whether you're talking about physicians or midwives. The best caregivers want to listen to you and will work with you.

Every single component of your ideal birth might not be accommodated for in that particular facility, but like you said, it's absolutely worth asking for.

The woman who came into Vanderbilt from my story had no clue she was going to need a cesarean, but she was in a place where she knew it was okay to ask those questions. Her question asking improved everything.

Sarah: I know you're really passionate about women receiving quality evidence based care and being cared for in a respectful way. Would you say that feeling 100% comfortable asking those kinds of questions with your provider is one of the most important things in all of pregnancy and birth?

Mavis: Yes, I would! I often have friends, or friends of friends telling me about their pregnancy and I hear this phrase lot ... *"I knew it didn't feel right. I knew I was in the wrong place, but I didn't want to change. I was afraid to change. I really thought he or she was a great doctor or was a good midwife or whatever, but it didn't feel right for some reason. I wish I would have done that differently."*

That really gets to me.

It's one thing to have a Cesarean and look back on it and be able to say *"Everything possible was done. I did everything I could have done. The people around me did everything they could do."* That's

120

ultimately what we strive to be able to say, versus hearing a mom say, *"Gosh, if only I had been allowed to do this, if only I'd been allowed to do that, if only these other people had done these things..."*

Oftentimes, that's *why* we have a much harder time recuperating after birth. Knowing that you and your birth team did *everything* possible during labor and birth will help you recover faster and transition you forward with your baby. It allows your mind to have closure on your birth. It allows you to move on.

Sarah: I've talked with hundreds of women who've felt that same way and who've actually said that exact same thing - they wish they would have spoken up! And here's what's so cool, when the same women were having their second or third babies, they did speak up. They assertively asked for what they wanted, changed providers, or whatever. And they found that their "fear of speaking up" was all in their mind. Once they spoke up, things changed.

The hospital staff or provider was happy to help and give them what they wanted or needed. They had no idea the mom wanted something different to happen. They didn't know something different was important to the mom, simply because the mom didn't communicate it clearly or assertively.

You suggest three things mamas can do to have a better pregnancy, labor and birth, what are they?

Mavis: The first is to absolutely speak up during your pregnancy and during your labor. If you want things to go differently than they are going, speak up. Speak up so you can understand all your options.

It's really easy to do, just like you're talking to your friend about something, just ask a simple question like ... "Hey *is there another way we can do this? I'd really like 2 more hours, can you give me 2 more hours? What if we tried this? What if we tried that? What if I did this? What if I did that?"*

It's so important to participate in your decision-making.

So many of us don't ask questions, because we have this fear that we're going to upset somebody and that somebody will take it out on us. Or they'll make us feel a certain way. And a lot of times we feel like we don't have the authority to ask questions.

That's a very vulnerable situation to be in. That's why people don't ask the questions.

As you said Sarah, we don't need to know everything about everything to ask questions. This is your baby, your body and your experience that'll be with you for a lifetime. So why not ask questions to get as much information as you need to feel more comfortable.

Sarah: The second thing you said is not to give birth on a battleground. What do you mean?

Mavis: It doesn't serve you or your baby well to labor and birth in an environment that feels like there's hostility around. And neither does it serve you well to have your husband fighting with the nurse or physician about the things you really would really like to have happen.

There's a really easy way to avoid this. Whatever you're choosing to have for your baby, make sure you've communicated your wants and needs way ahead of time, like during your prenatal appointments. Active labor is not the time to begin communicating.

Communicate early and often.

Sarah: The third suggestion you had was for mamas to find a way to trust in *their* ability to grow and birth their baby.

Sometimes that's not easy to do and is easier said than done. So how do we actually do that?

Mavis: It's definitely a challenge at times. And our culture is very technology focused, so there's a tendency to think that if we use all the technology possible, we'll have the best outcome possible during birth.

That's not necessarily so.

For each piece of technology offered to you [meaning each machine used, etc.] or automatically given to you, and for each intervention offered during labor and birth, step back and ask:

1. *Is this medically required?*
2. *What are the pros and cons?*
3. *With my situation and what I know, why would I do that?*
4. *Why wouldn't I do that?*
5. *Why do I even need that?"*

Ask questions about the things that are routinely done.

As far as the pregnancy goes, we only have a few babies in our entire lifetime. If you're like me, you only have one. But even if you end up having 6 babies, compared to all the experiences you'll have over your entire life, your births make up only a very small number of your whole life's experience.

And those experiences are precious.

So why not shape each one?

Why not be involved in the few experiences that'll have the biggest impact over your entire life?

Getting back to trusting our own capabilities to grow and birth our baby, every woman will find that trust in a different way. For some, spirituality will help them relax and trust. Other woman will have other ways to find that trust.

123

Every woman has her own birth story.

My birth is not your birth.

All of us have our own journey. We all have our own way of finding peace within ourselves from and during our different life experiences. I think that's a really key element for us to embrace during pregnancy. And if we can apply that during pregnancy, it will help guide us in birth too.

Sarah: Thank you Mavis for encouraging us to be involved in all of our journeys to the Motherland and to ask for things that may not be the norm. We improve our births and the health of our babies by asking more questions at every stop along the way!

Supporting Evidence

There was a review done of 53 studies in 33 different countries with, 554,568 participants. [xvi] All of this research looked at breastfeeding after c-section delivery. This review found that early breastfeeding rates were a lot lower in c-section deliveries than in vaginal deliveries. Most likely because hospitals don't allow their patients the opportunity to breastfeed until they are in recovery which can be an hour or more after baby is born. **With mamas who initiated breastfeeding early, whether they gave birth via c-section or vaginally breastfeeding rates were rock solid.**

Early breastfeeding is critical to breastfeeding success.

Regardless of what kind of birth you have, the sooner you get baby to latch on, the easier ALL of your breastfeeding will be.

You already know breastfeeding benefits last a lifetime. Creating an "early breastfeeding opportunity" for your baby is a worthwhile pursuit [for all the health benefits you get too!].

This study[xvii] published by the Padua University School of Medicine Department of Pediatrics, in Italy, looked at breastfeeding patterns in 2,137 newborns born full term. They found that mamas who delivered their babies via c-section had a lower breastfeeding rate (after being discharged, and followed up with at the seven day, three months and six month mark), than mamas who gave birth vaginally.

They equated a lower breastfeeding rate with the inability to comfortably breastfeed after delivery and in the postpartum period for c-section mamas.

But we're teaching you right here, right now, that the best medical research evidence says you can breastfeed right after a c-section. We're also showing you *how* to comfortably breastfeed after a C-section delivery, so you can breastfeed! You can do it!

Evidence Based Birth researcher, Rebecca Dekker, PhD, RN, found three randomized, controlled research studies on skin to skin 30 to 50 minutes after c-section and found that there were no adverse effects of doing skin to skin during this timeframe.

In fact, in one study[xviii], the average baby temperatures were higher in the babies doing skin to skin, than in those who didn't. In this case, higher temps are a good thing. It means the baby is starting to regulate its own temperature.

In another study[xix], one group of babies did skin to skin with their dads while mama was in the post-operation room. Those babies cried less and were calm and drowsy, more so than the other babies who were left in the bassinet.

Rebecca also found one study[xx] on skin to skin immediately after c-section (like 1 minute after). Babies were placed immediately on mama's chest for up to 5 minutes and then some of them got to stay for an additional 25 minutes, the others spent the next 25 minutes on daddy's chest. Then both groups got to do 90 more minutes with mommy. This study found no adverse effects from this skin to skin time after c-section and found that the babies who spent time with mommy breastfed a lot earlier (which increases the chance of breastfeeding success) than those who were hangin' with dad.

Another review of 34 randomized studies involving 2,177 mama-baby pairs found the exact same thing as the study above. Babies cried less, interacted with their mommies more, breastfed earlier and for a longer time and no negatives or risks were found to be associated with early skin to skin.[xxi]

One last little nugget I want to mention is according to the CDC's (Centers for Disease Control) website [xxii] just over 40% of hospitals report giving skin to skin for at least 30 minutes within one hour after an uncomplicated vaginal birth and just over 32% of hospitals reported giving women skin to skin for at least 30 minutes within two hours after uncomplicated cesarean birth. If you want to see how much skin to skin time hospitals give moms in your state, check out this link[xxiii] (look under the "most" column"). Nevada, you've got some work to do!

In Short

One good question could change the outcome of your birth.

And help to improve the birth of women and babies after you. Just like it did for that mama in Mavis's story.

That's the most important take away from this chapter. The best providers expect you to ask questions. They encourage you to ask questions. They want you to have the best experience possible. You're a team. You're in a partnership with your provider. You partner with them by asking questions. Have we mentioned how important it is to ask questions yet?

How to Get Skin to Skin After a C-Section

Download questions to ask and a summary of evidence here:
http://bit.ly/1g6ucjJ

1. Talk to your provider during your prenatal appointments and set the expectation that IF things should head in a c-section direction during labor, that you want skin to skin ASAP after birth (as long as all is well with mama and baby).

   Ask for their commitment to make that happen.

   If your provider doesn't commit, gives you a wishy-washy answer or says *"sure when you're in recovery,"* then it's time to educate them on the latest research and evidence showing how it's done. A lot of providers don't know the medical research evidence like you now do. Go to #2.

2. Hand the summary of evidence that you printed (from link above) to them and talk to them about all the benefits. Highlight the fact that there are no adverse effects to baby or mom and ask them to review the evidence you've given them. If they give you a solid commitment, ask if it's possible to set up another appointment (that will last 10 minutes) where you can talk to the anesthesiologist AND your provider together. You want to be crystal clear and know that your doctor will lead the charge and set expectations NOW for you and your baby to get skin to skin at birth and even if a c-section is required. Ask your anesthesiologist NOT to give you medications that will sedate you and make you out of it and super sleepy. You want to be as alert as possible. The rest of the plan is below.

3. You'll need two support people in the operating room with you. One to help facilitate the skin to skin and the other to take pictures and help with baby! Doulas are a great help, and as you're interviewing, ask them about their experience facilitating skin to skin during c-sections (just in case dad or another family member isn't available).

4. Make sure you're wearing only your hospital gown (no bra, or camisole or anything underneath) and that your spouse or birth support is wearing a button down shirt so he can do skin to skin if needed.

5. Ask them to put the EKG leads on in such a way that, you will still have plenty of space for baby (with no interference from monitors). Some nurses will surely say, "*I can't put those anywhere except in the middle of your chest honey, because that's just how we've always done it.*" Remember mama, you don't care how they've always done it, you care about doing

what's best for your baby, which is supported by the best medical evidence in existence! You're not making this stuff up, the leading hospitals and providers in the country provide this level of baby friendly and mother friendly care. Maybe your provider could even talk to someone at Vanderbilt to get comfortable with it. The point is this ... talk through this entire plan during one of your prenatal appointments and BEFORE the c-section.

6. Talk to your spouse and have them remind the nurses that instead of being brought to the warmer, if baby and mama are stable, you would like baby to be brought to mama ASAP. They can dry baby off on top of mom. Since this is probably not standard operating procedure, it's important for dad or birth support to gently remind them.

7. While your partner meets your baby and is bringing baby to you, have your doula or other birth support get your gown unfastened and ready for skin to skin. Your birth support should be ready to take pics!

8. Ask if your hands can be free, but even if they can't, just keep going with it. Have birth support help dad unswaddle baby and place baby horizontally across both mom's breasts, so baby and mama are chest to chest (and skin to skin), then have birth support cover mama and baby with blankets.

9. **One person has their hands on baby at all times** (to make sure baby is secure on mama's chest). Baby will probably start rooting around lookin' for mama's booby. If possible, situate baby so she can find what she's lookin' for. Mama may also be able to use her hands to help with this and stroke and touch baby. Baby is solely held in place by the spouse or birth support.

10. If mama starts to not feel well, have partner ready to take baby and do skin to skin instead. The button down shirt is handy here, and hubby will probably have scrubs on too. Scrubs can be cut quickly (it's no big deal to cut those, hospitals go through 'em like some of us go through hot 'n now Krispy Kreme doughnuts) to make room for baby on the chest. Staying near mom while doing skin to skin, if possible, will help her feel involved and will help her own oxytocin to flow.

11. Ask the nursing staff to wait until that golden hour (or two) is over before they weigh and measure baby.

**

It's interesting to me that when it comes to home renovations, we put everyone who'll be in charge of our renovations through their paces. We interview them. We look for reviews and references. We tell them exactly what we want, what we want it to look like, what we want the material to be, how we want them to do it. We communicate very clearly and purposefully with people who have some responsibility when renovating our house.

But then we have this total hands-off mentality and mindset when it comes to someone having a lot of responsibility with the most important moment of our entire lives, our baby's birth.

I don't get it. Do you?

And I was like that with our first baby and looking back, the reason why is because I didn't think any of my thoughts, feelings, insights and desires were worthwhile or valuable.

I didn't think they were valuable because I thought I needed a medical degree to make them have any sort of value. I thought they were just another of the many "crazy hormonal and emotional" thoughts from a pregnant chick.

Because I thought that, I started my first pregnancy by leaving *everything* in the hands of "medical professionals." That changed once I saw that my doctor's main interest was pumping me through his practice. He wasn't concerned how I felt as a woman or about birthing my first child.

So I broke up with him.

[I talked a lot about breaking up with him in my first book. It's called "Going to the Motherland: things to know for your journey."]

Thank goodness I found a new, incredible practice with providers who listened to every last question I could think of, who asked me questions like "how's work going?" and went out of their way to make sure I felt supported.

It's the same thing when it comes to c-sections. Don't just assume that whatever experience you were hoping to have before, has to go out the window because a c-section is medically required.

There's a good chance you can improve your c-section experience by talking it through with your provider. There are easy things that can be done to make your experience family-centered and to keep the focus on your baby's birth.

As Mavis mentioned, getting into a kerfuffle with the staff at the hospital will not serve you or your baby well. So knowing what you would like to happen and communicating that in a really nice, non-threatening way is all you can do. How they receive it and respond to it is up to them.

I know it sounds kind of silly, but that's why practicing what you say is actually a really good idea, it gives you a chance to prepare and think through what you want to say and how you want to say it, optimizing your chances for getting what you want. Because as you've learned, as soon as you can see your baby, the better. The sooner your baby can lay on your chest, the better.

You can have skin to skin after a c-section! The best research and medical evidence supports skin to skin after a c-section.

It's also a solution that'll increase your breastfeeding success. As long as mama and baby are doing well, the comfort and the nice distraction for mamas to have their baby nestled on their chest doing skin to skin, while surgery is being completed, will lead to more opportunities for immediate breastfeeding. Getting breastfeeding going right away helps baby kick start their life. They get that valuable "super food" colostrum and learn the "suck, suck, swallow, breathe" rhythm. It also gives mama much needed confidence and encouragement, that even though things may not have turned out as planned, bonding, breastfeeding and getting to know baby doesn't have to suffer.

Just like it doesn't (ever) occur to me to ask for a discount at Lowes on a refrigerator, it may not occur to you to ask for something to be done during a c-section that isn't "the norm." But now you know. So go for it mama! A lot of hospitals are starting to look at changing their policies. The best hospitals already are changing their policies, because they're focused on moms and babies. Some hospitals just need their customers to ask for it, so they can see the demand and respond by changing to a new "norm."

That's how progress happens!

If their response is not what you want, then press them to explain **why** their "no is a no." You can politely point to Vanderbilt University Hospital, which accommodated the request of one customer, and found that it was a great experience for all.

Vanderbilt is now a leading hospital in the US for doing family friendly c-sections. All it took was one mama to ask.

Just as it may not occur to you to ask, it probably doesn't occur to the doctors and nurses to offer a c-section that is "family friendly" and conducive to mama, daddy, baby bonding. Not because they are meanies who want it to be sterile and unpleasant for you, but because it just never crossed their minds that there's a better way to do this!

As long as mama and baby are both doing well, which, as Mavis pointed out, is usually evident fairly quickly after baby is born, there is no medical reason why skin to skin can't be achieved after a "normal", no complications, c-section in that first hour after birth.

Take Action

How to ask for skin to skin after c-section:

Here's the link to download a printable version
http://bit.ly/1g6ucjJ

1. Ask for it at your prenatal appointment, or if it's an emergency c-section, ask for it beforehand. Say something like this:

"Do you promote and encourage skin to skin immediately after baby is born?"

or

"It's really important to my husband and I that I can do skin to skin with our baby immediately after birth as long as baby and I are doing well."

If they say "no" then you ask:

"Are you familiar with the leading research and evidence that supports it?"

2.   If they push back and say they don't do it, protocol, etc, then ask them if you could try it one time, and print out the 11 steps to doing skin to skin after c-section. And show that you're willing to lead them through it because you're educated about this, confident and super prepared. You're ready!

Okay mama, are you ready to find out how simply waiting for two minutes might give your baby the biggest health boost of their lifetime? More miracles await! Let's dig into the next chapter.

Chapter 5

How Waiting 2 Minutes Can Improve Your Baby's Health For Life

with Dr. Sarah Buckley, MD, Author, Mom of 4

In two minutes, you can give your baby a health boost that'll last them their entire lives. It's the miracle of all miracles. It's the easiest preventative health boost they'll ever get. And it's backed by the best research and evidence from the leading medical institutions of the world. Many providers never talk about it, many birth education classes never even cover it (ours didn't and a lot of other moms told us theirs didn't either) and many hospitals don't do it.

This miracle will help your baby get oxygen during THE most important few seconds of their entire lives ... right when their lungs have to inflate for the very first time.

The boost will protect your baby from becoming anemic as they get older. It'll help your baby's brain develop. It'll give your baby extra stem cells, the super valuable cells which might help them avoid or beat a major disease later in life.

Here's the crazy part, there is no procedure is involved. It costs nothing. It only takes two minutes. And there are no adverse effects for your baby.

So how do you get this BIG super boost of health for your baby?

You do nothing.

For two minutes after your baby is born, you do nothing. I know, it sounds weird ... or gimmicky ... or fake ... or something ...

Nope. It's real.

It's been medically proven.

The most highly respected medical research centers in the world reviewed existing studies and have done new studies ... the results are clear.

Your baby gets a ton of clinically measurable benefits that improve their health for a very long time.

That's what this chapter is all about. We'll show you what this super health boost is and teach you how to get it for your baby.

Here's why we think you'll want to learn more about it- all of your baby's vital organs have to instantly "turn on" and start working right at birth (your placenta did all of the work while they were in utero). For all of those vital organs to work, they need an energy source (or they simply won't work). The energy source their organs need are huge amounts of oxygen.

Waiting two minutes to clamp your baby's umbilical cord gives them up to 33% more blood and more oxygen right at that acute time when their bodies have to have it to start working.

Or a better way to say it might be:

Waiting two minutes to clamp your baby's umbilical cord prevents them from being deprived of 1/3 of their entire blood supply during the most demanding few minutes their bodies will ever experience.

They've been using that blood for nine months. So many things have to happen for them to instantly transition to life outside the womb. More blood and more oxygen mean easier breathing and better functioning of their vital organs.

It can kinda make your head hurt but think about it this way: red blood cells carry oxygen to your baby's vital organs like the FedEx man carries Zappos shoes to your front door. Ya with me?

Dr. Sarah Buckley will share with us why delayed cord clamping vastly improves your baby's health.

We're also going to check out the actual evidence supporting delayed cord clamping, what the associated risks are, and what the standard of care is in most hospitals (standard of care means what is accepted as "best practice" by medical professionals, in other words, what they're actually doing). We'll talk about all the benefits to delayed cord clamping. But most importantly, we'll teach you how to get it for your baby.

From the chapter above, you already know who Dr. Sarah Buckley is. But in case you're reading this chapter first, we'll just mention that she's a mom to 4 kids and an MD in Australia, with a specialty in obstetrics and family planning. Dr. Buckley travels around the world educating moms, doctors, nurses and midwives about this very topic (as well as many others).

***

> "Delayed cord clamping is normal. It's just what's supposed to happen when we don't prevent it from happening."
>
> -Dr. Sarah Buckley

Sarah: So let's get right into it, what is delayed cord clamping and how does it happen in normal birth?

Dr. Buckley: If you've read my work, you know one of my foundations is understanding what other mammals do during birth and why. Other mammals don't clamp their baby's cord after birth. My friend said to me *"If we were meant to clamp our baby's cord right after birth, then we'd be born with a clamp on our thigh so we'd be ready to go."*

There's a reason why we don't have that clamp. Mother Nature designs the birth system so that in the minutes after birth, the baby gets a big influx of blood. We call it the placental transfusion. The big transfusion of blood comes from the placenta, because the placenta has been delivering the baby its blood while in the womb. The blood has sort of been stored in the placenta during those last minutes of birth. The placenta has been doing the work of many of the baby's vital organs while they've been developing and growing.

While in the womb, there are a lot of things the baby doesn't have to do. Sometimes I call it "Hotel de Womb", because everything is intact and done automatically for the baby.

Your baby doesn't have to breathe, your baby doesn't have to digest, your baby's kidneys and liver don't have to function, your baby's skin doesn't function for heat exchange either.

All of those vital organs are "on hold" while your baby is in the womb. Your placenta performs the work of those organs. Because those organs are "on hold" and are not yet working, they don't need blood.

But suddenly at birth, your baby's organs must immediately do all the functions they were meant to do and that the placenta was doing before birth. To instantly do all this work, your baby needs maximum profusion of their blood supply directed to their organ systems. Mother Nature designed this perfectly. That is exactly what the placental transfusion does, it gives your baby that extra blood, helping them transition and transition easier.

The blood comes to your baby over several minutes after birth (approximately between one and three minutes depending on the position of the mother and baby).

Here is how it works:

As the baby comes out, the cord is still attached to the baby and the baby's placenta is still in the mom's uterus (the uterus is the womb). The mom's uterus is still contracting, and every contraction squeezes the placenta. As the placenta is squeezed, it sends a push of blood into the baby. That push of blood increases the baby's blood flow. Then the uterus relaxes and a little bit of blood can even flow back. So there's a sort of step-by-step increase in the baby's blood volume.

As this continues for a few minutes time, the total amount of blood the baby gets is up to 33% more than if the cord was clamped right away. This is the baby's own blood. It's the blood they've been using during pregnancy. It's usually about one hundred mils. Depending on the situation, some babies might even get more.

It's a very significant amount of blood. It's a large amount of blood that your baby gets and your baby needs.

If we clamp and cut the cord right after birth, your baby doesn't get any of that blood. The clamp prevents any blood from getting to your baby. There is no placental transfusion possible.

If we wait, placental transfusion is possible. You could say your baby gets their blood volume restored.

Early cord clamping has been traditional or you could even say "historic." It was first done in the 1700s when women first went to bed to have their babies. Early clamping was said to spare the bed linen, because if you clamp and cut the cord right away, there is not much bleeding. I imagine it was a bit trickier to do back in the 1700s, but it was historical.

Sarah: Best for the linens, but not best for the baby.

Dr. Buckley: And then in the last 2 decades there's also been a misunderstanding about what happens when the baby gets a placental transfusion. There's been an idea that the baby can get too much blood.

That's not possible. The baby doesn't get too much blood. The baby gets just the right amount.

And we think now that the baby also regulates its own blood volume. Every minute of every day we're all regulating our own blood volume, because it's so important how much blood we have. We want just the right amount to near profuse all our organs, but not too much.

That's true for your baby who regulates their own blood intake during their placental transfusion. Some babies actually get less than a hundred mils, some babies get 60 or 80 mils and the most I've seen is a baby who got 164 mils, which was half the baby's total blood volume at birth! So it's a system that Mother Nature has devised so the baby gets exactly what they need. If we clamp and cut the cord, they can't get any of it.

Sarah: So to make sure everyone understands how fast this happens, let's talk about it as we'll actually experience it. Let's say you just gave birth, yay! You feel like *"Yeah! It's over, I did it! I'm exhausted, I wanna celebrate, I wanna sleep, I wanna hold and look at my baby"* all at the same time and then before you wipe a tear away … boom … your baby's umbilical cord has already been clamped and cut.

You won't even realize it's been done.

It's so fast. As in like 3 seconds fast. Just know how fast the opportunity can pass you by, if delayed cord clamping is something you're interested in. I didn't have a clue how fast this happened. I wish I did!

Ok, let's also talk about the umbilical cord so we're all crystal clear on why this matters...what all does the umbilical cord do?

Dr. Buckley: Sure, your baby's heart pumps blood through their body, then through their umbilical cord (umbilical arteries) and to the placenta, which is attached to the wall of the mother's uterus. And while their blood goes through the placenta, the placenta performs all those organ functions that I described earlier. The placenta oxygenates the blood. That's how the baby gets oxygen, because obviously they're not breathing while they're swimming in the amniotic fluid inside the protective amniotic sac.

The placenta also transfers glucose and nutrients to the baby, because the baby obviously isn't eating either. Then the placenta takes all the baby's waste away, because the baby's kidneys and liver aren't really working yet. The placenta also transfers heat away from the baby and to the mother, just like our skin lets heat off by passing it thru our skin. Well, the baby can't do that either, so the placenta acts as a heat exchange organ.

So the placenta performs all of those functions for your baby and then the blood comes back from the placenta at just the right temperature, beautifully oxygenated, with good nutrients and no waste and goes through the umbilical vein into your baby's body.

Your baby's body, the umbilical cord and the placenta are all part of your baby's circulatory system in the womb.

As the baby travels down through the mother's pelvis, there's a little bit of pressure on the cord. The tight quarters sort of squash the cord a little bit and the circulating blood gets a little bit blocked. When that happens, a little blood builds up in the placenta and then right after your baby comes through that tight squeeze in the pelvis, the cord releases. When it releases, the baby gets a large amount of blood right after birth (about 66 mils or so).

So if the cord is clamped right away after birth, the baby misses out on some or even all of that blood. I'll talk about the studies in a minute, but when we talk about *early cord clamping (ECC)*, we're saying within 20 to 30 seconds after birth.

Sarah: What does the best medical research evidence say about delayed cord clamping (DCC)?

Dr. Buckley: Delayed cord clamping is just normal. It's just what is supposed to happen when we don't prevent it from happening.

So that means if we clamp the cord immediately after birth, we're actually intervening during the normal birth process. That's why we say early or immediate cord clamping is an intervention.

And by intervening in the normal transfusion of your baby's blood, we actively stop that transfusion from happening. We've intervened.

If we clamp the cord early, the baby misses out on that 100 mils of blood. There are a lot of really good things in that 100 mils of blood. And as we'll talk about, there are a lot of stem cells in that 100 mils of blood. I'll describe what stem cells are and what they do.

But there are other critical factors in that 100 mils of blood, iron being a very important one. There are about 30 to 35 milligrams of iron, and that's equivalent to the iron in 100 liters of breast milk. That's one full month's worth of breastfeeding in that 100 mils of blood your baby would receive.

The baby who has the cord clamped early (ECC) will miss out on all those iron stores. That's the most compelling evidence we have, right now, for not doing early cord clamping, your baby will miss out on that iron.

Studies[xxiv] have shown that the baby is more likely to be anemic, to not have enough iron in their red cells during their early days. That means your baby will not have the maximum amount of iron stores available to them during their early weeks and months ahead. Iron is what your baby needs for their growth and development, especially for their brain growth and development. It is very significant for your baby to have an iron deficiency.

And while your baby is breastfeeding, there's only so much extra iron they can take in.

Another reason is that you want enough blood to transfuse all of those newly opened organ systems. So there's a possibility, in fact probably a strong possibility, that when the baby doesn't get that 100 mils of blood during delayed cord clamping that those organ systems are not so well profused. Some people even say that the baby's brain could miss out on a significant blood supply at that time after birth, which could be difficult.

Those things are not as well-researched as the iron component, but there are lots and lots of other very helpful reasons, that your baby will miss out on, should they not get all of their own blood from the placental transfusion.

Sarah: Cord blood has stem cells, red blood cells and white blood cells. White blood cells are germ and infection fighters, so it seems like it would be really beneficial to have 30% more germ fighters in your body as a little baby.

Dr. Buckley: Yes, that's true. And the red blood cells are particularly beneficial, because red blood cells have hemoglobin, which carries oxygen. So the baby misses out on a lot of oxygen carrying capacity in the early days and weeks, because it takes several months to build up more blood cells.

In addition to what you mentioned Sarah, there are other factors that we're beginning to understand about the baby's cord blood. Your baby gets some protective and healing factors, like neuroprotector factors for example, because Mother Nature expects, to some extent, birth to be a stressful process. There are

144

factors that heal tissue damage, there are factors that heal brain cells, and there are factors that nourish the brain cells.

So there are a whole lot of things in that cord blood, during the placental transfusion, that are designed to optimize your baby's transition into the world. And that is no surprise, babies have been doing this for millions of years. Mother Nature has worked out what babies need for optimal survival.

Sarah: What does the evidence say about the risks associated with delayed cord clamping?

Dr. Buckley: It was once thought that babies would get too much blood, that's supposedly the reason why they clamped and cut the cord right away. But if you go back and look at the studies that were done, they were poor quality studies. They didn't even use "normal" babies at term in the studies. I think that we can say the evidence of risk for delayed cord clamping is pretty much nonexistent.

There's no evidence that delayed cord clamping is harmful.

Something that has been talked about is that the baby might get too much blood if drugs are used, so maybe I need to talk a little about that. So what generally happens for babies born in an institutionalized setting and some babies born at home, the mother gets what is called "active management of the 3rd stage."

"The active management of 3rd stage" has three components and they're usually all still used. The 3 components to actively managing a mother's 3rd stage of birth are:

1. Early cord clamping
2. Administration of an oxytocic drug, which is a drug that makes the uterus contract. In the US it's called Pitocin or Syntocinon and some places use Misoprostol.

3.   Pulling on the cord after birth to get the placenta out.

Those are the 3 components and they're generally all done together as a package. And they're done as a package because of some evidence that supposedly says that this prevents postpartum hemorrhage for the mother.

So it's a bit ironic, we're trying to stop the mother bleeding but at the same time we've been forcing this hemorrhaging at the baby through early cord clamping. We're starting to think that maybe it's not such a good idea to do early cord clamping for the baby. They're looking at this whole package and pulling apart each of the three components to look at them more closely.

Now we're thinking maybe the oxytocic drug is useful, but the other two components, the early cord clamping and controlled pulling on the cord to get the placenta out aren't really necessary.

So the oxytocic drug causes the mother's uterus to contract, and if you remember how I said it's the mother's uterus contracting that pushes blood to the baby. You could imagine that if a uterus is contracting more strongly because of this drug, than that could push too much blood to the baby. Does the baby get too much blood if we don't clamp the cord while we're giving the mother this oxytocic drug? That's been the reason for the concern.

There's not a lot of research on this. But my non-research based opinion is this ... if we believe the baby's physiology regulates their own blood volume (as all humans regulate their own blood volume) by controlling the to and fro of the cord blood for their final blood volume, then we'd have to conclude that if the baby gets too much blood, they can send it back.

In fact, it was very interesting that one of those studies showed that when the baby cried, the baby actually sent blood back to the placenta. If we believe that, then as long as the cord isn't clamped, the baby still has the ability to regulate its own blood volume. Personally, I don't believe giving the oxytocic drug is going to be harmful. It probably speeds up this placental transfusion. Rather than taking 2 or 3 minutes it probably takes 30 seconds, but in the end, as long as we don't clamp the cord preventing the baby from getting the amount of blood they need, the baby is going to get exactly the blood volume that is perfect for their own biology.

Sarah: Wow, it's amazing how our bodies were designed!

Here is a quote dating back to 1801. The quote comes from Erasmus, he was the grandfather of Charles Darwin. He said, *"Another thing injurious of the child is the tying and cutting of the naval string too soon, which should always be left till the child has not only repeatedly breathed, but till all pulsation in the cord ceases. As otherwise, the child is much weaker than it ought to be, a portion of the blood being left in the placenta, which ought to have been in the child."*

Erasmus knew this in 1801. Birth hasn't changed. This is nothing new.

If there aren't any serious risks, and your baby will get up to 33% more blood, plus all the other benefits that is supported by research, why isn't this the standard of care by every provider, in every birth setting (hospital, birth center and home birth), for every baby right now?

Dr. Buckley: Yes, it's a little shocking isn't it? Certainly there has become a fashion for intervention in childbirth in many areas over the years. And this specific intervention was well intentioned, because postpartum hemorrhage is the largest cause of maternal mortality worldwide. A lot of women die from postpartum hemorrhage in poor countries. That usually happens because they start off with marginal nutrition and then they can't afford to lose their blood.

So we do really want to protect moms at birth. The intention of this "active management package" was to prevent excessive bleeding, but we hadn't really looked at each component critically. That's why evidence based care is so critical for every mom and baby.

There's a group in the UK called the Cochrane Collaboration and they do studies, look at the evidence and make recommendations for specific areas in healthcare. It was set up by a man called Archie Cochrane and he gave obstetrics the proverbial wooden spoon, because he said obstetrical practice was the area least supported by the evidence.

Obstetric providers have not been good at looking at the physiology, looking at the evidence and practicing according to what it says.

[This is why we work so hard to bring you evidence based info in easy to read and learn ways friends … you deserve it!]

So I think we'll see the recommendations change to delayed cord clamping in the coming years, I have no doubt about that, and not only for healthy babies, but for babies that need resuscitation at birth.

We talked about what Erasmus Darwin knew, and women and midwives around the world knew this too, for many, many years. If the baby is weak at birth or is not doing well at birth, the baby particularly needs 100 mils of blood. There is actually a practice called "milking the cord," which means squeezing the blood out of the cord until the baby gets that full amount of blood.

There's a fantastic paper written in the British Medical Journal, whereby the author says that if the baby needs resuscitating, wait

148

one minute. In that minute, the baby can get a large increase in their blood volume that could auto-resuscitate the baby. They effectively could resuscitate themselves with that extra 100 mils of blood.

Sarah: Let's move to what situations would prevent delayed cord clamping. When would delayed cord clamping not be beneficial for my baby?

Dr. Buckley: In general, the physiology works, so delayed cord clamping can be the default position during the physiological 3rd stage of birth. I'd say for 99% of babies, delayed cord clamping is going to be beneficial. There are very occasional risks, when a baby is growth retarded for instance, that the baby doesn't have a large circulatory volume. It may or may not work in an instance like this, but I think I've got to say the default position is that delayed cord clamping will be beneficial for your baby.

Not clamping the cord at all is actually what I recommend. All the additional blood your baby gets will be better for your baby.

Let's go back again to what other animals do. No animal ever clamps the cord. They don't do anything until the placenta comes out. That's what we're designed to do, we're designed to do nothing until the placenta comes out.

And of course I'm not recommending we chew threw the cord like other animals do. But there's just no medical benefit or need to do anything until the baby's placenta comes out. Once the placenta is out, we can clamp and cut the cord however we want.

What generally happens physiologically is that the cord clamps itself. The vessels in the cord start to clot and close up and you can generally cut the cord within 15 or 20 minutes after birth, there's usually no bleeding. So we don't even need to clamp actually.

Sarah Blight: Interesting, I didn't know that! Let's move on to our last point, which is … *"I want to have delayed cord clamping and I'm giving birth at a hospital. What do I need to do to get that?"*

Dr. Buckley: You need to talk to your caregiver. You need a caregiver that is approachable, open-minded and ideally one who has read the research themself. You want one who knows the evidence and benefits of delayed cord clamping.

You've got to really have an honest discussion with your caregiver and say what you want.

And I recommend showing your caregiver the research and evidence, show them the benefits of delayed cord clamping by showing them the studies. For example, the International Federation of Obstetricians and Gynecologists (FIGO) and the World Health Organization recommend delayed cord clamping. There are papers published in major medical journals on this as well.

Sarah: If you have a physician who doesn't really know the research, can you give it to them?

Dr. Buckley: Yes, you can and you should. That's exactly right. Just one more thing to say about finding the best caregiver, when you have these conversations with your caregiver, you'll know right away how open and willing they are to having this kind of discussion with you. If they are, that's a really good sign. When you approach your caregiver with something that is important to you (that's based on the latest research and evidence mind you), it is a very telling litmus test.

If they say, *"oh well, you know, I don't know about that"* or *"I don't think so"* and they're not willing to look at what you want, and that's based on research evidence, then that's pretty telling about how they will most likely be at your birth.

To be honest, if they're totally closed about delayed cord clamping, then I recommend you find another caregiver.

If they're closed-off to providing you and your baby the best evidence based care, what other evidence based best practice are they closed-off about or are they unwilling to provide moms and babies?

What's going to happen in the operating room or in the birth room? Even if you clearly say that you want a specific kind of evidence based care, are they going to go against your direction, go against the evidence and intervene anyway?

And I have another suggestion on how to get delayed cord clamping, even if you are in a position where it doesn't seem like you can get it for your baby and you don't have any other options (because the hospital won't support you, a nurse isn't listening, or your doctor isn't open to it) …

…I'd recommend you take on delayed cord clamping as a spiritual practice.

Some people say and believe the "essence" or "spirit" of the baby comes into the baby right after birth. And the truth is that the baby actually does receive a lot of genetic information through that cord blood.

So here's what I recommend you do … I recommend that you take on praying over the baby immediately after they're born. But before you go into labor, say to your caregiver …*"I don't want the cord cut until our prayers have stopped."* And then you make sure those prayers take a very l...o...n...g time!

Sarah: This is such a great tip!

151

Dr. Buckley: There's another spiritual practice to consider if you decide delayed cord clamping is important to you. It's called lotus birth.

Lotus birth is where you don't actually clamp the cord at all.

You don't use a clamp and the baby is attached to the umbilical cord and the placenta until the cord drops off the baby at their umbilical. The benefits are obviously all the benefits we've previously talked about, plus you can lie completely still and be in the moment. Another benefit is that you just miss a whole lot of drama after the baby is born.

You miss the drama about clamping and cutting the cord, pulling the placenta out and completely avoid the drama about taking the baby away to get weighed, measured, and all those things that can absolutely wait. The drama can easily interfere with those important and magical first moments you'll never have again with your baby.

Mother Nature designed those moments for the mother and baby to meet for the first time, look deeply into each other's eyes and fall in love. That's Mother Nature's blueprint, that's what our baby's and our own physiology is wired to do.
That's what is meant to happen.

That's what will happen unless we allow all this fussing around to distract us from giving our baby all these proven health benefits. So you might want to look into lotus birth as kind of extra-delayed cord clamping.

Sarah Blight: To make sure we're all on the same page, 'cause I didn't know ANY of this when Jackson was born, let's talk in specific terms about how long we're supposed to "delay" during delayed cord clamping. From talking with other doctors and midwives, my understanding is that we should delay clamping

the cord until the cord itself stops pulsating. The reason we clamp the cord only after it stops pulsating is because that's when all the beneficial cord blood has completed its transfer into the baby. Is that right?

Dr. Buckley: Great question! Most providers will clamp the cord in about 30 seconds or less. Delayed cord clamping (DCC) basically means "waiting longer than most providers would ordinarily wait," because there is no one "right time" to delay, so long as you are satisfied with the placental transfusion your baby has received. So I would say anything longer than 30 seconds you might call "delayed."

But a better question to ask might be this ... "What are our bodies physiologically designed to do? What's going to best optimize our baby's and our own physiology?

I think your answer is the same answer we've said several times ... the way to optimize your and your baby's physiology and health is to do what other animals do. And that means we do nothing until the placenta comes out.

That's my definition of a truly optimized physiology for mom and baby after birth.

Now, some people say *"yes, the best time to clamp the cord is to wait until the cord stops pulsating."* The reason why they consider this to be the best time to clamp the cord is because the baby's heart pumps blood through the vessels while the vessels are still open. A pulsation of the cord is a visual representation of your baby's heart pumping blood through those vessels that are still open. When those vessels close, the cord stops pulsating. The thought here is that the baby has transferred all the beneficial cord blood.

But there is still a little bit of blood and oxygen exchange that is possible thru the veins, which doesn't pulsate. So even when the cord stops pulsating, that is not necessarily the mark of a finished placental transfusion.

That's why I recommend waiting until the mother births the baby's placenta.

The most important thing you remember and take away is this ...

There is no hurry!

Mom and baby can be skin to skin. No one can take the baby away for any reason. After the mother births the baby's placenta, then you can clamp and cut the cord if you like. That's my recommendation because it optimizes the physiology for baby and mom.

Let me be clear about one thing, anything beyond 30 seconds is going to be beneficial to your baby. Think through this information we're talking about now so you can decide how long past 30 seconds you want to go with your baby.

Sarah: This is such important information Dr. Buckley, thank you for sharing all of your experience, knowledge, insights, opinions and for highlighting the evidence! You're such an inspirational doctor, woman, mom and we're honored to have you included in this book!

Supporting Evidence

Researchers[xxv] looked at 15 randomized, controlled trials which compared early cord clamping to delayed cord clamping. There were 3,911 mama-baby pairs. In the delayed cord clamping (DCC) group, they found that the babies had significantly higher birth weights (which makes sense if they have up to 33% more blood in their bodies), and they had higher hemoglobin concentrations than the early cord clamping (ECC) babies. Remember that hemoglobin's job is to transport oxygen through the blood.

ECC babies were less likely to be treated for jaundice, which we will talk more about further down. They were also found to be twice as likely to be iron deficient at 3 to 6 months of age, than the babies who had DCC. Iron is critical for healthy development of the brain, central nervous system, etc. Babies' bodies need iron to make hemoglobin (hemoglobin carries oxygen to all of our cells)- see evidence here.[xxvi]

There was another analysis[xxvii] done of 15 randomized, controlled, studies which involved 1,912 newborns. Delayed cord clamping was done 2 minutes after birth and early cord clamping was done immediately. Researchers also found in this study that DCC done to full term infants had benefits continuing on through infancy, including a reduced risk of anemia (deficiency of red blood cells or hemoglobin).

This analysis found that there was an increased risk for DCC infants to have polycythemia, which is when bone marrow makes too much red blood cells. But researchers stated that this condition appeared to be "benign."

Researchers did note that as many as 60% of the fetal red blood cells in circulation between baby and the placenta are found in the placenta and that this blood is super rich in hematopoietic stem cells. These stem cells are being studied a lot right now because they are able to form other kinds of cells like muscle, blood vessels and bone.

An article in the Journal for Cellular and Molecular Medicine published in 2010 made a good point: organ systems continue to develop and mature in babies after birth. What happens then if these awesome, rock star stem cells aren't allowed into our babies' bodies? The authors state that *"the artificial loss of stem cells at birth could potentially impact later development and predispose infants to diseases such as chronic lung disease, asthma, diabetes, epilepsy, cerebral palsy, Parkinson's disease, infection and neoplasm."* (Note: neoplasm is the abnormal growth of tissue, a characteristic of cancer).[xxviii]

If you're like me and you're thinking: *"But the benefits are sooo amazing of delayed cord clamping and it doesn't cost anything besides a couple minutes, so what am I missing? Why in the world don't more providers do delayed cord clamping?"*

You are not alone.

Researchers wonder the same thing.

Doctors and midwives who practice DCC as a standard part of their care wonder why their doctor and midwife counterparts don't practice what the evidence so clearly says to do.

So what in the heck are the attitudes of OBs towards delayed cord clamping?

They sent a survey to OBs representing 43 practices in the UK, US, Canada, Australia and other European countries. They had a 100% response rate and found that 53% did delayed cord clamping only occasionally, 37% did it never. Unawareness of the benefits of delayed cord clamping was the reason that half of the non-compliant respondents gave for why they don't do it. [xxix]

But the main reason doctors said they don't do delayed cord clamping was "difficulty with implementation in clinical practice."

Insert crickets chirping.

Explain to me how doing nothing for 2 minutes qualify as "being difficult?"

Honestly, as a mother of 2 children, doing nothing for 2 minutes sounds like a slice of heaven!!

If this doesn't smack us women across the face and make us realize we need to start hiring and firing our provider based on their ability to actually care about practicing medicine based on medical evidence, then I have no idea what will, ya know?

Finding a provider (or firing the one you have) who cares enough to give us evidence based care minimizes our and our babies' risk during pregnancy and birth.

This is exactly why one of our YourBabyBooty mantras is ... "There's a gap between what the best science says and the maternity care most of us women actually get."

I'm not going to lie mama, when I was researching and came across that phrase "difficulty with implementation", I got all kinds of fired up. Steve had to bust out his mad soothing skills cause I couldn't get to sleep after that!

In Short

Remember that guy named Lance Armstrong? In case you have no idea who I'm talking about- he's the cyclist who won the Tour de France seven times- one of the hardest physical, endurance races in the world. And that dude won seven times.

Lance has since received a lifetime ban from the sport after he admitted to doping. Turns out, Lance ran one of the most sophisticated blood doping operations in the history of sports.

So what in the world does this have to do with your baby? Hang with me.

According to the investigation[xxx], Lance would use certain hormones to boost his production of red blood cells and oxygen intake. This increased the amount of oxygen being delivered to his muscles. More oxygen meant more fuel for his muscles, ultimately giving him much higher performance, faster recovery and better endurance.

Science proves that the more red blood cells you have, the more oxygen gets to your organs and muscles, and the better your body performs.

Alright, let's forget about Lance and other athletes who've used this tactic to optimize their body for high performance.

Your baby's body needs these same red blood cells for its own high performance during their demanding transition into this world! Your baby needs a big time oxygen boost way more than some dude riding a bike up a mountain.

This is a matter of getting your baby's organs more oxygen right when they have to instantly all start working for the very first time.

It's almost comical that we are hanging out in the hospital, with nowhere else to go and nothing else to do, and yet there's an urgency (to save a whopping 2 minutes) to get the cord clamped and cut, baby weighed and measured, and the nurses on their way stat, when all the research clearly shows that allowing your baby an extra 1 or 2 minutes, before clamping the cord, will give them a slew of clinically measurable benefits and lasting health improvements (and it's FREE!).

Benefits like 33% more blood, with more red blood cells carrying oxygen to all their newly working vital organs and more hematopoietic stem cells that will strengthen their bodies. Can you imagine how long it would take and how much it would cost to develop a drug (or procedure) that would give your baby all those benefits? It'd be insane. Unless we stop it from happening, all those benefits happen in just 2 minutes time and cost a hefty zero dollars.

A better question might be … why would your provider or you ever consider early clamping the cord (ECC)?

Isn't it kind of a no-brainer?

Cutting the cord right away is a practice born out of habit, not out of evidence based practice.

Jaundice

One of the risks of delayed cord clamping is jaundice. Let's refresh ourselves on what jaundice is. Infant jaundice is when the baby's blood has extra bilirubin. Bilirubin is the yellow colored pigment of red blood cells. Jaundice is common in babies especially those born before 38 weeks and even in breastfed babies.

Here's how jaundice happens …

The baby's liver isn't quite yet able to get all the excess bilirubin out of the bloodstream (and this all is making sense to you now that you know about all the miracles happening in your little newborn's body after birth and the fact that your baby's liver hasn't even had to work actively until birth, it's primarily been a storage place for sugar and iron), so the excess bilirubin makes baby's skin and eyes yellow.

According to Mayo Clinic[xxxi], treatment often isn't necessary for mild jaundice, 'cause the liver will get going and take care of the extra bilirubin itself.

Other treatment options for jaundice include putting baby in the sun for 15 minutes a day. We did this with Jackson after he was born. He was very jaundiced. We just stripped him down to his cute lil diaper and put him next to us on the couch in a nice sunny spot. He caught a few sun rays and sure enough, in a few days his jaundice cleared right up.

Other options are light therapy. Similar to putting your baby in the sun, light therapy works because it's a special light that changes the shape of the bilirubin molecules so that your baby's body can get rid of them when they poop or pee.

The point is that Jaundice is treatable. **It's not a risk that outweighs all the other benefits DCC gives your baby (according to the best research and evidence available).**

Should I Get Active Management or Go Au Naturel After Baby is Born (the 3rd Stage of Labor)?

Dr. Buckley mentioned 3 ways that providers "manage the 3rd stage of labor" to prevent postpartum hemorrhage in mamas:

1) Early cord clamping

2) Administration of an oxytocic drug which makes the uterus contract.

3) Pulling on the cord after birth to get the placenta out.

We've thoroughly discussed why early cord clamping (ECC) is not evidence based practice and Dr. Buckley talked very quickly about making the uterus contract with oxytocic drugs, like Pitocin, as being effective to stop mama from hemorrhaging. Then she briefly discussed pulling on the cord after birth to get the placenta out.

Let's dig into this for a moment just so you understand what this pulling on the cord thing is all about.

According to Dr. Buckley, in her book "Gentle Birth, Gentle Mothering: a Doctor's Guide to Natural Childbirth and Gentle Early Parenting Choices", Francois Mauriceau, a French obstetrician, first recommended gently pulling on the umbilical cord to get the placenta out in 1673. It was thought that the uterus would close before the placenta came out.

Basically pulling on the cord after birth is also called "controlled cord traction." The provider has one hand providing traction on the cord, and the other hand is doing counter-pressure on the lower abdomen. This is done only when the provider is sure that the placenta has separated from the wall of the uterus. It's also done in conjunction with giving the mama Pitocin (or other oxytocic drug) to help her uterus efficiently contract.

This research study[xxxii] looked at 24,293 mamas giving birth in 8 different countries. All the mamas were given oxytocic drugs. Half of the mamas delivered their placentas using their own effort, i.e. contractions and gravity and the other half had controlled cord traction to get the placenta out. This study found that there was no increased risk of hemorrhage in the mamas who delivered their placentas using their own effort.

If you don't do anything and let your placenta come out on its own, it can take 10 minutes to an hour. Our midwife actually encouraged me to breastfeed our daughter right away so that my uterus would contract, which lessens blood loss and also starts the process of separating the placenta from the uterus. So this is one option if you're not keen on having Pitocin to "help" you with this part of your labor.

If you have chosen to have your provider help your placenta come out, you can expect it to take anywhere from 5 to 20 minutes.

If you're thinking *"ohmygosh, I thought once baby came out, I was done!"* I thought that too at first, but most of us are so entranced, snuggling and looking into their baby's eyes and enjoying our skin to skin time, that we don't really remember this part of labor.

Yay for that!

Delayed cord clamping is something that Steve and I never, ever heard of before our son was born. We didn't learn about it at our birth class and never talked about it with our provider. We hadn't heard anything about it. We just didn't know. We have no idea if delayed cord clamping was even done with Jackson.

Looking back, it seems crazy that some of the most important information that can help our babies live healthier lives is never taught by many birth classes or talked about with moms by the providers they've hired.

That's why we're here.

For you.

That's why we do our Easier, Healthier Birth podcast, our website YourBabyBooty.com and write the Birth Book series.

We're here to change that and to help get the invaluable experience, wisdom and evidence out and into your hands, so you can confidently make the decision that is best for your family. There's no right way to birth a baby, but there's a right way for you!

Risks and Benefits of Delayed Cord Clamping

Benefits	Risks
Up to 33% more blood for your baby	Jaundice (not considered a serious risk & is easily treatable)
More red blood cells which carry oxygen More white blood cells which fight off disease, bacteria & viruses	Polycythemia (when bone marrow makes too many red blood cells- researchers found this to be harmless)
More hematopoietic stem cells -strengthens immunity	
Less likelihood of anemia	
Awesome Iron stores through 6 months old improving brain development, etc.	

The World Health Organization (WHO) said in 2007 "The first minutes after birth are a very vulnerable period for both mother and newborn. The care that is provided during this time is critical to ensure not only their immediate survival but also their longer-term health and nutrition." [xxxiii]

So that's our job mama, to make sure out baby gets the best evidence based care immediately after birth. It helps them thrive at birth and long into the future too. You have an awesome toolbox of info mama to do this job easily and awesomely. You've got this!

Take Action

Simply tell your provider you'd like delayed cord clamping. And we explain below exactly how to do this, and some common objections from providers (and how to respond to them).

Top 5 Provider Objections to Delayed Cord Clamping & How to Respond:
*You can download a printable version by following this link:
http://bit.ly/KnJExY

1. *Your provider might say … "Delayed cord clamping takes too much time, my practice is just too busy."*

   Your Response: "Nearly 1/3 of my baby's blood is still in the placenta and umbilical cord after birth. The benefits of:

   - Up to 33% more blood for my baby
   - More red blood cells which carry oxygen to my baby's vital organs

- More white blood cells which fight off disease, bacteria & viruses
- More hematopoietic stem cells -strengthens immunity
- Less likelihood of anemia
- Awesome Iron stores through 6 months old improving brain development, etc.   and the fact it will only take a few minutes. Don't you agree all these clinically measurable benefits for my baby's health are worth 2 minutes of your time?"

2. "Immediately clamping the cord prevents severe postpartum hemorrhage."

Your Response: "Actually, research doesn't support that. A 2009 Cochrane review[xxxiv] of 5 trials including 2,200 mamas found that there was no significant difference between early cord clamping and delayed cord clamping as far as postpartum hemorrhage or severe hemorrhage. You can check it out here.[xxxv] "

3. "Healthy babies born at term don't get benefits from delayed cord clamping."

Your Response: "Studies don't show that to be the case at all. It doesn't matter when baby is born- they all receive the benefits of delayed cord clamping. In fact, babies that receive delayed cord clamping have a much easier time transitioning after birth and efficiently pumping blood to their organs and their lungs to breathe. Plus, the concentration of fetal stem cells is at an all-time high after birth. These stem cells help organ systems grow and develop. Depriving my baby of these beneficial stem cells *could* predispose him/her to diseases like chronic lung

165

disease, asthma, diabetes, epilepsy, cerebral palsy, Parkinson's disease, infection and neoplasm.[xxxvi]"

(The point here is that we're just beginning to understand ALL the benefits and there are no significant risks. This statement by any provider is simply not supported by any medical evidence.)

4. **"Delayed cord clamping can lead to jaundice."**

Your Response: "You're correct, studies show that there is an increased chance that delayed cord clamping will lead to jaundice. According to Mayo Clinic, treatment is often not even necessary for mild jaundice. Once the baby's liver gets acclimated and starts functioning fully (which will happen more effectively when delayed cord clamping delivers more oxygen and more blood to my baby's organs), it's no problem. If the jaundice is more severe, light therapy and even putting baby in the sun for a few minutes each day will help. The benefits of delayed cord clamping far outweigh the potential risk for jaundice, according to the best research and evidence. Wouldn't you agree? [xxxvii]"

5. **"You can't do delayed cord clamping and skin to skin because gravity will reduce the flow of blood from placenta to your baby."**

Your Response: "You have a point, gravity is a factor. But the only influence gravity has is how long the placental transfusion actually takes. If baby is on my chest doing skin to skin, it may take longer for the placental transfusion to complete, but it will still happen.[xxxviii]"

The point here friends, is that nothing your provider might say, trumps what the best research and evidence says. All of the research and evidence says delayed cord clamping will help your baby in measurable ways. And unless there is some severe problem with baby (like they need to operate right away, etc.), there is no reason why you can't have delayed cord clamping for your baby (even with a c-section, etc.)

How to Talk to Your Provider About Delayed Cord Clamping:

"Excuse me Dr. _____, but I just read the latest research evidence in the Journal of Pediatrics that it's best to delay cord clamping by 2 minutes and that means I would like to receive my baby on my chest and keep my baby there for at least an hour. I'm sure that you would agree with me that this is the best thing for neurological development and the enhancement of breast feeding and bonding."

If your provider pushes back on doing delayed cord clamping, you and your partner and birth support can let them know that you have spiritual intentions, you can say something like:

"Dr._____ or Nurse_____, we have a spiritual practice that is really important to us. Right after baby is born, we will need to have a spiritual moment (prayer time). Please respect this time and wait until we are done to proceed with whatever you need to do."

Or you can say:

"Dr. _____, this is a spiritual practice for me, I need to know that you support it. We would like for you to wait until we are finished with our prayer time before you do anything, including cutting the

cord after baby is born. Please place our baby on my chest and give my partner and I, a couple moments. Thank you for respecting our beliefs."

This is your time with your baby. If you decide you want delayed cord clamping, you'll need to actively make sure you're getting it!

***

Alright mama, let's go onward, shall we? The next topic we tackle goes hand in hand with delayed cord clamping and it was actually really hard to find any existing information that wasn't completely biased one way or the other. So we are here to be the voice of reason in the midst of the storm. We are Switzerland, completely neutral and presenting facts. You ready?

Chapter 6

Should I Consider Cord Blood Banking?

with Dr. Sarah Buckley, MD, Author, Mom of 4

Will cord blood banking save my baby's life?

Most of us have seen them, all the ads we're bombarded with. Then we get the pamphlets in our swag bags from the baby superstores after we register and flyers in the mail.

Am I a bad mom if I don't do it? Am I just being too cheap by not spending thousands of dollars to do it? But most of all, is it true? Is there anything to it? Is there evidence to back up the claims of all the benefits by all these cord blood banking companies?

If you're asking these questions, oh mama, you're not alone.

To be completely honest, I wasn't up to navigating through this maze when I was pregnant. But I always had that unsettled feeling that comes with not being educated and wondering if I was being taken for a fool, or missing out on the most incredible opportunity.

There's a lot of scrutiny surrounding cord blood banking. Who offers the service, how much does it really cost, how is the cord blood taken and how is it stored? When do we need to decide if we're going to do it or not? What about donating to a public blood bank? What should we consider to make the most educated decision for our babies?

Dr. Sarah Buckley is back.

She'll help us understand this important info, plus I did some good old fashioned investigative work to put all these pieces of the puzzle together. It's important to see what science really says about the possibilities of cord blood banking and what research says about how effective it really is at treating people. At the end of the day, this whole enchilada boils down to "did someone get better because of the banked cord blood?"

We think it's a better idea to make educated decisions based on research and facts rather than emotion. And quite honestly, fear. So lets get to it and get to the bottom of this topic of cord blood banking. Ya ready?

***

"Cord blood banking is like an insurance policy.

You're asked to shell out a lot of money for something that you may never need.

On the other hand, if you need it, you'll be glad you did. "

-Sarah Blight

Sarah Blight: What is cord blood banking?

Dr. Buckley: To understand cord blood banking you need to understand what normally happens to the baby at birth. In the minutes after birth, your baby has about 2/3 of their blood in their bodies and about 1/3 of their blood is still in the placenta (which has been in charge of delivering clean blood and oxygen to baby).

We covered this in the previous chapter, but let's review. Several minutes after birth, the baby's remaining blood in the placenta (up to 33%) automatically transfers to them. We call this the placental transfusion.

Mother Nature designs and intends for that blood to go into the baby. It has enormous benefits for our babies. Iron for example, in the few minutes after birth, your baby gets iron stores equivalent to the iron in about 100 liters of breast milk or an entire month of breastfeeding. And of course they get stem cells, the baby needs their own stem cells.

Cord Blood Banking companies paint all sorts of very emotional pictures about how beneficial it's going to be for babies and you'll only get this one chance to do it. And yes, it could help.

But really the chance of the baby needing or using that blood that you bank after birth is very, very small. Some people say 1 in 1,000, and that's the best-case scenario I've ever seen. Some people say 1 in 20,000 or even lower, and even if we're talking about 1 in 1,000, that really only means the chance of the baby having a condition that the cord blood could be used for. It doesn't mean the cord blood would be the best treatment for that condition.

If you look at cord blood banks' use around the world, there are very, very, very few uses of that cord blood for that particular baby that's autologous. Autologous means going to the baby itself. In fact the biggest use of cord blood banking is to siblings, to a match sibling.[xxxix]

Sarah: I want to make sure everyone knows why cord blood is considered so valuable. I don't want to make assumptions, because I didn't know this stuff when I was first pregnant. The cord blood has master stem cells (stem cells are valuable because they can renew themselves and have the ability to turn into many different types of cells, whereas non-stem cells can only stay as that type of cell that they already are), red blood cells (deliver oxygen and remove waster) and white blood cells (germ and infection fighters).

Dr. Buckley: The stem cells that are in cord blood are called "hematopoietic stem cells." After the baby is born, these stem cells are designed to migrate to the baby's bone marrow and begin to form these white blood cells and red blood cells, etc.

Those cells are very useful because they help your baby get more oxygen, fight off diseases, etc. And those are the cells that are taken away and banked.

Sarah Blight: Fear is a strong motivator. As moms, we start seeing ads that make us think and feel that the only way to ensure that we'll have a healthy child and healthy family later in life is to pay for cord blood banking.

When I was pregnant, I would see these ads showing a beautiful kid frolicking around some grassy field, blowing bubbles with his sister, smiling, giggling and having fun, and of course their dad is frolicking too. The ad asks if I want a happy healthy family?

Of course I do!

The message goes something like "If you want a kid who can frolic and be happy and healthy just like this kid, then the only way to ensure that it happens is to buy our cord blood banking services."

Feelings are powerful and marketers in every area of business tap into peoples' feelings to promote their products. I get that. But I'd rather know what the medical evidence says, not what the marketing department says.

Dr. Buckley: The main way that cord blood is used by the private cord blood banks and the public cord blood banks (which are like libraries- people donate their baby's cord blood and those needing blood search for a match for their own child) is to give people or children a source of blood when they need to repopulate their own blood cells.

A common example would be treatment for leukemia. The drugs given for leukemia basically kill the blood cells made in the bone marrow. And after those blood cells are killed off, you need to repopulate those blood cells in the bone marrow.

Generally, the standard of treatment has been to repopulate those blood cells from that child's own blood. So you take out the child's blood tissue from the bone marrow, they are treated, then the blood tissue is put back in. When their own blood tissue is taken out and put back in, there is obviously a 100% match for that child because it's their own.

Using another person's blood tissue might be an option. But if you put in someone else's bone marrow it has to be a good match, otherwise the body will reject it.

Cord blood acts the same way, it has to be a good enough match or the body will reject it.

For example, if you have a child who has leukemia, you could try and find a good match from your own bone marrow, from a sibling's bone marrow, or from a different child's cord blood taken at birth. But there's no guarantee. You don't know if the cord blood taken at birth will be a good match for their sibling who needs it. That is an example when cord blood banking would be most useful. You bank the cord blood taken from the baby's umbilical cord at birth, in case you might need to try and match it sometime in the future.

All the other uses for cord blood are very speculative. I'm not sure if they're still advertising this, but one company said it could save your baby from Alzheimer's. These are very, very speculative suggestions.

Ways that Cord Blood is Being Used Currently & Potential Uses in the Future

	Current Uses	Still Being Investigated
Diseases	Hematologic (blood disorders): -Acute Leukemia -Lymphoma -MDS/MPD (diseases where bone marrow makes too many white blood cells) -Inherited and acquired bone marrow failure syndrome -Hemoglobinopathies -Immune deficiency -Metabolic diseases -Solid Tumors	Non-Hematologic: -Cerebral Palsy -Diabetes -Hearing Loss -Immunotherapy for infectious disease or against tumors -Gene therapy -Autism
Source	Cord Blood	Cord Blood Umbilical Cord Placenta

Based on info gleaned from Haemotologica, the Hematology Journal.

Sarah: Also I want to add that scientists and researchers aren't completely sure if the stem cells being banked (even if they are an exact match) are as beneficial as fresh stem cells from other sources. Only time and more research can determine that. And that comes from Dr. Svendsen, a leading authority in stem cell research.

Can you walk us through an example how the cord blood would be taken?

Dr. Buckley: Sure. Let's look at it from the perspective of the cord blood bank. We want to get the most cord blood possible, because generally you're going to get more stem cells when you collect more blood.

The blood is usually collected from the vessels in the umbilical cord with a needle. The blood is usually collected into a special bag.

You're probably not going to get 100 mils, you may get 30 mils, 40 mils, or maybe 50 mils of blood if you're lucky.

GOOD TO KNOW...

Each cord blood bank has their own minimal amount of cord blood they can bank. The numbers I heard (first hand) from 4 of the major cord blood banks was anywhere from 10 mililiters to 40 mililiters as a minimum amount that can be collected from an umbilical cord.

***

Sarah: How long does the blood stay "good and usable" in the bank?"

Dr. Buckley: That question is difficult to answer because some of these treatments are new, and as I said some of the companies are new. But what we know is that a public cord blood bank generally guarantees the blood for something like 15 to 20 years and public blood banks generally have a lot of resources and they've been doing storing blood for a long time. The quality controls are extremely important for whatever blood bank you go with. For the blood to last a long time, the temperature controls must be very consistent and precise.

Personally, the other thing to consider is that at the moment, this is one way to get stem cells for research and treatments. But there's a huge amount of money being put in all around the world to find other sources of stem cells, and they've found stem cells in breast milk for example.

And if they can fiddle with the genetics a little bit, they could get stem cells out of their own cells as well.

I've just got to mention that when you sign up, if you sign up with a care provider (your OB or your midwife), ask them *"Are you being compensated monetarily or any other way if I sign up?"* because a lot of cord blood banking companies have compensated providers in the past. You need to know that as you make your decision. They should be declaring that they actually have a conflict of interest by signing you up and getting paid by the cord blood banking company.

I had a long and interesting dialogue with an executive from a cord blood banking company who offered me *"the more people you sign up, we'll give you 50 dollars for each person you sign up"*. There is a lot of money involved in this industry. If it costs several thousand dollars to initially take and store the blood, then several hundred dollars every year after to store the blood ... that's a lot of money. So you just want to know the full story if this is something you're going to consider.

Sarah: Why would we ever want to consider donating the cord blood to a public blood bank instead of paying to have it stored at a private blood bank?

Dr. Buckley: When you donate to a public cord blood bank, there's a much greater chance it will be used. The chances of you needing it for your own child, are so small (the figure I quote in my book is 1 in 15,000), there is a much higher chance someone else can actually use the cord blood. So, there is a very small chance of you needing to use it and it's a very large amount of money to bank it privately. Donating the cord blood to a public bank is a very generous thing to do, because it'll be someone you don't know whose cell types are a match and who will use that blood to help them in major ways.

Sarah: Thanks Dr. Buckley for this really solid info! We appreciate all you do for pregnant women all over the world!

Supporting Evidence

The Journal of American Pediatrics published an article that surveyed pediatric hematopoietic cell transplantation physicians in the United States and Canada. There were 93 doctors who responded (out of the 152 eligible ones) representing 9 transplants where the child used their own cord blood (autologous) and 41 transplants where the cord blood came from someone else (allogenic).

The physicians' summarized conclusion was this (as of 2008, when this article was written): very few transplants had happened from cord blood (from donors with no known disease or illness) being stored just "in case" something were to happen to that donor (the baby).

The ability to use autologous (stem cells collected from and then used for the same person) cord blood depends on the disease and what alternative stem cell sources there are. And in the words of the article, *"Few pediatric hematopoietic cell transplantation physicians endorse private cord blood banking in the absence of an identified recipient, even for mixed-ethnicity children for whom finding a suitably matched unrelated donor may be difficult."*[xl]

Scientists have been looking at how long cord blood can be stored and still keep its effectiveness. Several scientists, from the Department of Microbiology and Immunology at the University of Arizona, studied cord blood cells that had been frozen in liquid nitrogen for 7 years.

They found minimal effects on cell viability, the composition of the cell and the capacity of the hematopoietic stem cells.[xli] Another set of scientists, from Institute of Haematology and Blood Transfusion, Department for Cryopreservation in the Czech Republic, studied cord blood that had been cryopreserved (in liquid nitrogen) for 15 years and came to the conclusion that no damaging effect was found on the cord blood cells.[xlii]

According to an article written in the Hematology Journal, Haematologica[xliii], of the 500 patients who received cord blood transplants from family, 91% have had a 4-year survival (they had non-malignant diseases) and 56% survival (malignant diseases). This same article says that family directed transplants (or transplants done using family cord blood) do have advantages over getting a transplant from a non-relative: higher likelihood of survival, decreased graft versus host disease (GVHD), and bone marrow cells can be re-collected from the donor if there's a relapse or rejection.

We wanted to get to the bottom of this rumor floating around that it's not possible to do both delayed cord clamping and cord blood banking after birth. So I called five major American private cord blood banks and this is what I found out:

Out of the five I called, I talked to four of them. Out of the four I talked to, three said without hesitation that *"yes, it's possible we can do delayed cord clamping and cord blood banking"* and one said *"we don't recommend it."*

One of the companies that said, *"yeah mamas can do both"* also went further and said *"we encourage our families to stick with their birth plan and do the delayed cord clamping for however long they desire."*

This company also connected me to one of their genetics counselors who is a clinical specialist in cord blood banking and she said while they don't have any scientific evidence, they do have anecdotal evidence from doctors who report that they are able to retrieve sufficient cord blood even when mama does the delayed cord clamping. Of course each baby and cord are varying sizes and have different amounts of blood.

The company which said they don't recommend delayed cord clamping in conjunction with cord blood banking mentioned research that shows early cord clamping (ECC) isn't all that bad, as anemia and jaundice are the only "side effects" and that those are "treatable" conditions.

Since we know what the research evidence says, I pressed the company on this. I asked *"well what about babies starting life without 1/3 of their blood? Wouldn't all those red-blood cells and oxygen be significantly beneficial for baby at birth? Wouldn't these stem cells be super useful to them at birth?"* The representative responded that the company had not given him that kind of information.

Once I let him know that their competitors were accommodating mamas' desires to do both delayed cord clamping and cord blood banking, he asked me to send him any research and information I have on the topic. I sent him several research studies that show the benefits of delayed cord clamping. From talking to them more, it sounds like this company will be changing their recommendations soon.

In Short

Public vs Private Cord Blood Banks

In 1991 the first public cord blood bank was established in New York, since then there have been more than 100 public cord blood banks which have done 25,000 cord blood transplants (between unrelated people). There are accrediting agencies and governmental bodies that are in place worldwide to make sure that the cord blood collected from the public and donated to these public banks are legit and meet the standards.[xliv]

Private cord blood banks, on the other hand, do not have to be licensed in the United States and accreditation is voluntary.

Here's a fact, Netcord has established guidelines and standards for public banks in countries throughout Europe, Australia and Canada and offers accreditation (as does the American Association of Blood Banks), to private cord blood banks, but few private cord blood banks in the U.S. have voluntarily become accredited through them.

It is free to donate cord blood to a public bank, but you can only do so if you're giving birth at a hospital that participates in a cord blood collection program. This is definitely a great question to ask your hospital.

Private blood banking costs anywhere from $1,700 to $3,000 for the initial collection including the first year of storage and then $125 to $200 a year after that for storage. With private blood banking the cord blood is yours and can be used if and when someone in your family needs it. It's important to note that the cord blood may not always be a match with the person in need, even within the family.

How Much Does It Cost
for Different Private Banks?

We went to the websites of 3 large, private cord blood banks and jotted down their pricing. Then we estimated what it would cost to bank it for 20 years (since that's the longest that cord blood has been banked to date)- just to get a better idea of what it could really cost.

	CBR-Cord Blood Registry	Miracle Cord	Via Cord
Collection & first year of storage	$1995	$1995	$2250
Yearly storage	$130	$125	$125
20 years of storage	$2470	$2375	$2375
Total	**$4465**	**$4370**	**$4625**

It's no wonder people look in wild -eyed wonder when the words "cord blood banking" are mentioned. As I mentioned in the intro, just before Jackson was born, I had crossed off the last items on my to dos, every drawer and closet had been cleaned and organized and the freezer was full of food. We thought we were ready and then he came 3 weeks before we anticipated. I remember this feeling of panic as I thought about cord blood banking, because I kept putting off researching it. And now I know why! It's a freaking jungle out there!!

Using cord blood in transplants is incredibly new. [xliv]In fact, the first documented successful case was in 1988. A 5 year-old boy with a blood disorder received the cord blood from his sister, from when she was born.

There is no quality research (in other words, research that's not funded by cord blood banks, or conducted by physicians with vested interests in cord blood companies, or people who are opposed to it altogether) on this topic, which makes the jungle pretty dense, but not completely impassable.

Let's make like Nancy Drew (if you don't know who that is, you're making me feel really old right now) and put the pieces of this puzzle together and solve this mystery. Starting with the facts:

What we know about cord blood banking:

1. The amazing abilities of hematopoietic stem cells is continually being discovered and documented by research.[xlvi]
2. It is possible to do delayed cord clamping AND cord blood banking with most private banks.
3. Private cord blood banking can cost anywhere from $1,700 to $3,000 for the initial collection including the first year of storage and then $125 to $250 a year after that for storage.
4. Cord blood collection is harmless for baby and mother (as long as delayed cord clamping is permitted).
5. Family-directed cord blood transplants (when the cord blood is donated and used within the same family) have benefits over using cord blood from a public bank- these include a higher chance of survival, decreased "graft versus host disease" and the opportunity to recollect bone marrow cells from the same donor in case of rejection or relapse.[xlviixlviii]

6. The AAP, American Academy of Pediatrics discourages storing of cord blood at private banks for later personal or family use as a general insurance policy.[xlix]

7. American Congress of Obstetricians and Gynecologists' (ACOG) position on cord blood banking at private banks is that it has no position. It does recommend that physicians disclose that there is *"no reliable estimate of a child's likelihood of actually using his or her own saved cord blood later."* And that physicians need to disclose that it's unknown how long cord blood can successfully be stored and to disclose if they have any financial interest in the cord banking company.[l]

8. The Journal of American Pediatrics published an article which concluded that private cord blood banking for a child who has no known disease is not recommended.

9. Private blood banks are not subject to the same regulatory standards as public banks. It is voluntary.

10. As years go by, scientists are discovering more and more about what these stem cells, found in cord blood, can do. There are still a lot of questions about cord blood collection, methods of storage and how long they can usefully be stored, that are still not completely known.

11. There have been successful stem cell transplants, using stored hematopoietic stem cells.

Let's wrap all this information up in a pretty little package with a nice, awesome bow that would make Martha Stewart proud.

Cord blood banking is like an insurance policy.

You're asked to shell out a lot of money for something that you potentially may never, ever need to use. On the other hand, if you need it and it's for a close family member and they're a perfect match, or your donor needs it- you have it.

I spoke to my hairdresser about this issue, she was pregnant with her second and she said without hesitation that she was going to be banking her baby's blood because her nephew has a medical condition that could drastically benefit from these amazing hematopoetic stem cells. It was a no brainer for her and her family. She was happy to spend the money on the potential to help her nephew.

Your fears, hesitations, concerns, and experiences are unique to you. The thing you have to figure out is if you're okay with spending thousands of dollars to bank stem cells, which statistics say you'll probably never use. If you're cool with that, then you have your answer. If you're not cool with it, then you know your answer too.

The bottom line … there is no clear chart we can make for you showing you "if you bank your baby's blood, you can do this, and this, and this, and here are the limitations."

There is TONS of research and money being poured into cord blood banking right now. A lot of testing is being done. You have to decide, based on the current information available, if it's worth it for you and your family.

Take Action

It's time to figure out if this is something you'd like to pursue. So how do you do that? We can help you. Here's the old fashioned Pros & Cons chart. It's for you to fill in with your spouse. We've added some things to think about. Download this worksheet by putting this link in your browser: http://bit.ly/1lFy50c

	PROS	CONS
Private Cord Blood Banking		
Public Cord Blood Banking		
Neither		

1. What is the medical history in your family? Are there any known diseases that genetically you or a loved one could be susceptible to?
2. Will you feel a peace of mind?
3. How much is that peace of mind worth to you?

Questions to Ask Your Provider About Cord Blood Banking (private & public)

*These questions can also be downloaded
http://bit.ly/1giA7T0

1. Do you recommend cord blood banking? Why?
2. Is the hospital where I will deliver, part of a public cord blood collection program?
3. What is your experience with private cord blood banking?
4. Do you recommend any specific bank?
   a. Why?
   b. Are you paid by these banks?
5. If we decide to do delayed cord clamping, and blood banking, do you see any problems with that?

Questions to Ask Private Cord Blood Banks

1. How is the cord blood collected?
2. What are your special techniques to assure that you get the most cord blood possible?
3. Is it possible to do delayed cord clamping and bank cord blood with your company?
   a. Why or why not?
4. What is the minimum amount of cord blood you will bank?

5. What if the collection is not suitable? How do we get our money back?
6. How much is collection & banking per year?
   a. Does the price change with the amount collected?
   b. Is there a guaranteed price on yearly storage? How long?
   c. Do you have any discounts or promotions?
7. How does the cord blood get from the hospital to your lab- where is your lab?
8. How can we be sure that the cord blood we donate will not get mixed up with someone else's?
9. What security is in place to protect the cord blood while it is in the liquid nitrogen?
10. What about natural disasters? Do you have emergency plans in place?
11. Are you accredited? If so, with whom?
12. What process do we need to go through if we need to retrieve our cord blood?
13. What happens if we can't afford to pay for storage or we just decide we don't want to?
14. Can we tour your lab? (If we're in the area)
15. What assurances do we have that your company will still be here in 20 or 30 years?
16. In the event that the company folds, are we able to transfer our cord blood to another bank?
17. Do you have any guarantees?

Chapter 7

Does My Baby Need Eye Ointment Right After Birth?

with Rebecca Dekker, PhD, RN, Mom

Your best friend just gave birth and you are dying to see pics of that cute little bambino. She finally texts you one, you look at it-then enlarge it to get a better look. Super cute baby, but what in the world is that in her eyes? Why in the world does baby girl have vaseline in her sweet little eyeballs?

That shiny stuff that looks like vaseline is actually called erythromycin. It's eye ointment. And we're about to dig in and find out what the best research and evidence says about putting this stuff in our baby's eyeballs after birth.

The first questions that come to mind are: Is it necessary? Why? Is it medically proven? What are the benefits or risks of using that goop and honestly, what is it anyway?

To help us get answers to these questions we have Dr. Rebecca Dekker. She has a PhD and RN, and an Advance Practice Registered Nurse, APRN, is an Assistant Professor of Nursing at a major research university, is the founder of Evidence Based Birth. Dr. Dekker is an expert researcher and writer on evidence based healthcare. In addition to all of that, she's also a wife and mama to 2 kids.

Dr. Dekker has researched erythromycin and is here to teach us what the best research and evidence says.

> "Informed consent contributes to your well- being because you're an active participant in your healthcare and the whole process."
>
> -Rebecca Dekker, PhD, RN

Sarah: How did we start using erythromycin for newborns? What is the history?

Dr. Dekker: It actually has its roots in the 1800s. In 1881, there was a doctor named Dr. Crede, and he realized that infants in his hospital nursery were catching an eye infection during vaginal delivery. So he put two and two together and realized that infections were caused by gonorrhea, which is a sexually-transmitted infection.

So he put a compound called silver nitrate in the eyes of newborns, and in fact, during the first 6 months he started using the silver nitrate, the number of cases of newborn eye infection in his hospital went from about 35 cases per year down to 1 case. This became known as the Crede Treatment Prevention.

If you look on people's birth certificates, like I even saw my dad's from the 1930s, they'll say "Crede Treatment" showing that they put the silver nitrate in the baby's eyes. It became very widespread quite quickly, because they realized it was so effective at preventing this infection. It was like a pink eye, but a dangerous kind of eye infection, because it was caused by gonorrhea and about 3% of babies who caught this eye infection became permanently blind.

Sarah: You mentioned gonorrhea and that's obviously a sexually-transmitted disease. Was that the only way babies were getting the eye infection, by contracting it, through their moms, during birth?

Dr. Dekker: Gonorrhea is not as common in the U.S. anymore. The main cause of this type of pink eye now is chlamydia, which is also a sexually-transmitted infection. So both gonorrhea and chlamydia can cause this type of severe pink eye that can lead to permanent eye damage or blindness. These are pretty much the only known causes of the permanent eye damage from this kind of pink eye. So we know that this dangerous pink eye comes from chlamydia or gonorrhea.

Sarah: Is it possible for babies to contract this if they're being delivered via c-section or only through vaginal birth?

Dr. Dekker: The only way for a newborn to catch this is if their mom is actively infected with chlamydia or gonorrhea. So if the mom does not have chlamydia or gonorrhea, then the baby can't catch it.

But it's also thought that it's impossible for a c-section baby to catch it, if the mom's water never broke. Let's say it was a planned c-section and the mom's water never broke, then there was no pathway for the infection to get to the baby's eyes, so it's thought that it's impossible for that baby to catch it.

Sarah: And that's because when the baby is still in the amniotic sac, the sac is a completely sterile environment?

Dr. Dekker: Correct. There have not been any reported cases of this happening in that type of situation.

Sarah: Okay, got it. So we're all on the same page, chlamydia or gonorrhea cause the actual eye infection, and the eye infection itself has a crazy name … it's called ophthalmia neonatorum.

Dr. Dekker: Yeah, ophthalmia neonatorum. That is a type of pink eye that occurs within the first month of life, and it's caught at birth.

Sarah: How do you actually know if you have chlamydia or gonorrhea, what symptoms will we see?

Dr. Dekker: Well, that's the thing, most people who have chlamydia or gonorrhea do not have any symptoms.

So most people who have it, don't even know they have it. Anyone who's sexually active can catch chlamydia or gonorrhea. Some people are at higher risk. There's some areas of the country, some areas of the world where rates of infection are higher.

You can definitely avoid both of these conditions if you're in a long-term mutually monogamous relationship, you know your partner is not infected and you've also been tested.

You're at higher risk if you have multiple sexual partners or if you're under the age of 25, but like I said, most people don't have any symptoms, so they don't know that they have an infection unless they're screened.

Sarah: Okay, I've heard the following scenario a lot from women ... "I know I've been in a monogamous relationship for a long time. I know that I don't have either of these STDs, but I'd still like to have this erythromycin eye ointment for my baby because I'm worried about staph infection or some kind of other infection." Is that a myth or is there some truth to that?

Dr. Dekker: I've been hearing that a lot. A lot of moms are telling me that nurses are telling them, "*well, you don't have a sexually-transmitted infection, but your baby will catch a staph infection if you don't use this ointment.*"

The pink eye or conjunctivitis can be caused by lots of things. Babies and grownups can get pink eye from viruses, from bacteria, from chemicals, from blocked tear ducts. Both of my babies had that, they had very small tear ducts and would get pink eye because of it. So there's lots of things that can cause pink eye. The dangerous one, the dangerous pink eye that can cause blindness is caused by chlamydia and gonorrhea.

A staph infection or a bacterial pink eye can be treated really easily with topical antibiotics. And saying "*we should give every baby eye ointments for that staph infection*" would be like saying "*we should give every kid in elementary school eye ointment once a week to prevent staph infection.*"

This doesn't really makes sense, because first of all, there's never been any research or evidence to show that giving eye ointment an hour after birth will prevent a staph infection.

It would be very easy for your baby to catch a staph infection a couple days later, simply because staph bacteria are everywhere. They're all over the hospital. They're all over our skin. So it's always possible for a baby to catch a bacterial eye infection and giving them eye ointment at birth isn't going to necessarily prevent that from happening. Does that make sense?

Sarah: Yes, that makes total sense. Let's move on and learn what the research and evidence says about using erythromycin to prevent this ophthalmia neonatorum or let's just call it "the dangerous pink eye."

Dr. Dekker: One way we can prevent the dangerous pink eye is to give all newborns an eye treatment to prevent the infection from happening. This is called prophylaxis and it means you are doing something ahead of time to prevent something bad from happening. And right now, using eye ointments in newborns is recommended by lots of different organizations including American Academy of Pediatrics. It's also mandated by law in many US states.

But when we look at the research evidence, there have been 8 studies that kind of semi-randomly assigned people to get different treatments to prevent dangerous pink eye, and they found that erythromycin was much better than silver nitrate at preventing the chlamydia type of pink eye.[li] But the studies that we have are of poor quality. Those studies are what we call randomized trials, which are the gold standard, but they're not good quality randomized trials.

If you look at some really large studies, where they looked at lots and lots of people, and there's one really important study in

South Africa where they weren't using any eye ointment. There were like 273 cases in 100,000 births before they started using the eye ointment. Then after they started using the eye ointment, the number went down from 273 to 34 cases out of 100,000 births.[lii]

So there is some evidence that eye ointment does prevent the gonorrhea and chlamydia type eye infection pink eye, but the important thing is you know there are other options as well.

Sarah: Okay we will move on to those other options in a sec. Right now, let's talk risks and benefits because with any medication or any procedure, there'll always be risks and benefits. What are the risks and benefits to using erythromycin?

Dr. Dekker: Evidence suggests that erythromycin can lower your baby's risk of catching the dangerous pink eye from chlamydia or gonorrhea, and to me, it's actually helpful in areas where rates of chlamydia and gonorrhea are really high, for example, in Africa and in certain parts of the United States as well.

It's also fairly cheap. It probably costs less than a dollar to put on babies.

It can also be helpful if you don't know what the mom's health has been like, meaning if she doesn't know she's infected or not.

On the other hand, what are the potential harms of this medication? We do know that eye ointment, erythromycin, can cause eye irritation and blurred vision.

There have not really been any studies that show that it interferes with bonding, but it's possible that it could, and it is uncomfortable for the baby, and it's not 100% effective.

So you can give erythromycin eye ointment, but you can still catch the dangerous pink eye. It's not going to work 100% of the time. And there have been drug shortages where a couple years ago, we didn't have enough erythromycin in the United States, and healthcare workers started using different eye ointments that had never been tested in newborns, and they found out later that some of these were harmful to the newborn.

Sarah: Yikes, that doesn't sound like a very good idea. This leads into my next question which is, when we're presented with options as parents and we're not sure, we're kind of trying to weigh our options, and figure out what we're doing, a really great question is always "what other options do I have" or "can I opt out of this?" So let's start with that first question, as parents, what other options do we have instead of erythromycin?

Dr. Dekker: Well, that's a good question because back in the 1880s, when they first started using the silver nitrate for human baby's eyes, there really weren't a lot of options, but we have options now.

Back in the 1880s, they didn't even have antibiotics yet, so if a baby caught an eye infection, there was nothing you could do about it.

Also, some things have definitely changed since a lot of these laws were passed requiring the use of the eye ointment. For example, most women are now screened for sexually-transmitted infections in pregnancy, and they're treated with antibiotics if they have them.

So the benefits of being screened are that if you do have an infection, it'll be detected and you can get treated, and that will improve both your health and the health of your baby.

So that's one option, get screened for chlamydia and gonorrhea. The drawbacks to getting screened are that no screening test is 100% perfect, so there is a slight possibility that you could be positive for say chlamydia, but the tested said you were negative. So that's a slight possibility.

Another option, and this is what they use in England and a couple other countries like Australia, is to just wait and see if the baby gets the dangerous pink eye. And if they do, then you treat your baby with antibiotics. That's an option that wasn't available back in Dr. Crede's time, but is available to us now.

Most of the time, if that happens, the baby would need systemic antibiotics, not just any antibiotics in the eye, but antibiotics that they take orally or by IV. And in some countries, but not in the US, there's another option called Povidone-iodine. That's a disinfectant drop that you can just drop in the baby's eyes. It's very cheap, it only costs a couple of pennies. And the studies have shown that it's very effective at preventing the dangerous pink eye, but it's not available in the US. So that's not an option here.[liii]

Sarah: I'm guessing that asking you why, (if it's so effective and so cheap, isn't it available here in the US) might be a whole other conversation.

Dr. Dekker: The FDA approves which medication can be used and marketed in the US, and they want a US study. There have been studies done in lots of other countries, but the FDA wants one done here, and the cost of doing that study isn't worth the time of the big pharmaceutical companies, because like I said, the medication only costs pennies. So there would be no point in them paying for a big study to approve this medication that they wouldn't make any money on. So it's mostly for financial reasons that we don't have that option.

Sarah: It's very important to understand "Informed Consent" during labor and birth. It's super important because it gives you the freedom to make the decisions you think are best for your baby. Informed consent allows you to use all your options you have during labor and birth- there is no one right way to birth a baby, but there's a right way for you.

Specifically, during the golden hour or when deciding about the eye ointment, informed consent is what enables you to opt out of the eye ointment, if that's what you think is best for your baby.

So can you explain in detail exactly what it is and why it's important to moms as they labor and give birth?

Dr. Dekker: Sure! Informed consent is basically a process. It's a process of communication where you as the patient or as the person who is receiving health care, you are enabled to make an informed and voluntary decision about whether or not you're going to accept something or decline something.

This is both an ethical concept and a legal concept. The ethical side has two major parts, if you're giving informed consent, it means: 1) That you understand what you're consenting to or not consenting to, and 2) That you're freely able to consent.

So, in the first part, understanding means that you've been given adequate and accurate information about your situation and the different treatment possibilities, including the option of no treatment, and you've been given this information in a way that you can understand, meaning the language style, and on a level that you can understand [as opposed to, for example, only being told about 1 option instead of all 3 options, or being talked to in medical speak quickly and then that provider rushes out the door and you're left to make a decision without fully understanding the situation or all your options].

In other words, in order to be ethically valid, your consent has to be informed. You have to know what's going on.

And that second part of informed consent means that it's freely given and that you have a voluntary choice. You're able to freely tell someone "yes" or "no" without being coerced or unwillingly pressured by other forces.

Sarah: So why is this so important for moms?

Dr. Dekker: I would say it's good for your health because informed consent helps protect you against treatment that you don't want, that you might consider harmful or that you might consider unnecessary. And informed consent contributes to your well-being because you're an active participant in your healthcare and the whole process.

Sarah: So this doesn't just apply to pregnant, labor and birth, but anytime we're getting or our kids get medical care?

Dr. Dekker: Exactly, it definitely applies to all kinds of healthcare.

Sarah: So how does this work together with certain treatments being mandated? Let's use erythromycin as the example. Let's say I'm a parent who's done my research, I know I can't possibly pass along the dangerous pink eye to my baby because I've been in a monogamous relationship, or I've been tested and tested negative. I've weighed the risks and benefits and have determined that I don't want to give my baby medication in their eyes when it's not medically required ... how does that play out?

Dr. Dekker: There definitely has been a tug-of-war between informed consent and the concept of public health, and there are some other ethical obligations that may override the requirements to get informed consent. For example, if there was a strong claim for the "good" of public health, limits could be set on what you're allowed to choose or use. This tug-of-war has been going on for a long time.

Back in 1902, there were a lot of people dying from small pox in Massachusetts and the public health department required people to be vaccinated. This one man named Mr. Jacobson refused, and he was actually tried and convicted in the state court for not getting vaccinated.

200

In a lawsuit after that, it was called Jacobson versus Massachusetts, the judge basically said that the community has some right to protect itself against an epidemic of disease that threatens the safety of people. And so that was one example showing how informed consent can be overridden to protect human good.

But you still have this other principle in informed consent, just 10 years later in 1912, the Supreme Court heard a case where a woman was operated on against her consent, and the justices basically ruled that every human being has the right to determine what's done with his or her body.

So you've got these two things, this right to informed consent, this kind of right to determine what's to be done with your body, and then you've got this concept of public health. And these things can clash sometimes.

But the problem with erythromycin is that it's not really an emergency public health issue anymore. And we also have other options, whereas when they passed all these laws mandating the use of erythromycin in the early 1900s, there weren't other options and we didn't have antibiotics. We didn't have screening.

Now we have a choice, the treatment might not be necessary and it might not do anything for the health of your own baby, but it's still seen as a public health issue. It's still the law in many states.

So we have this problem where all these state laws are still hold the same standard from over a hundred years ago, that all babies should be treated with eye ointment even though we have other options now.

Sarah: So in those states where it's mandated, and assuming you're in the hospital environment, can you even opt out? Or will your baby be getting erythromycin no matter what?

Dr. Dekker: Even in a home birth setting, like in New York state for example [home birth is legal in New York state], which probably has the strictest state laws I've seen, they basically come out on their Department of Public Health website and say parents do not have the right to refuse erythromycin eye ointment at a home birth. So the home birth midwives are required to administer the ointment, or they have to lie about it or they can lose their license kind of thing.

I think it really depends on what your options are in your state. And it depends on how much you want to rock the boat, because I think a lot of women will say "well ... it's state law, it's really not that harmful, and it can cause some eye irritation, but that's the only really bad effect, then I'll just let them put the ointment into my baby's eyes, even though my baby doesn't need it, because I don't want to rock the boat." A lot of parents just don't want to make waves, and the risks aren't really that big to this medication, so I can see them making that decision.

On the other hand, some parents may feel really strongly and moved that "this medication is unnecessary and I don't want it done to my baby and I live in a state where it's mandated." In that case, they have to be ready for a battle if the hospital where they're giving birth is enforcing that state law.

Sarah: So it's important to check with your provider, because they're your go-to person, they're your team member. Hopefully, they're a valuable team member who is educating you on all of these decisions, what the laws are and what all your options are. That's why asking "what are all our options" is worth its weight in gold.

Dr. Dekker: Yes, definitely talk with your care provider. But there are a lot of myths out there. Some care providers will say "oh, it's state law," but then if you actually go look at the state law on the public health website for that state, it's not law.

So you really want to do a little bit of research and find out what the law is, so you know what you're dealing with … ask your provider, you can call the labor and delivery floor at your hospital to ask, you can look online at your state laws and look at the newborn procedures to find out exactly what your state law says.

It you want to decline, it might not a big deal for you to decline at all. You may just have to sign a waiver. Worst-case scenario, some hospitals are afraid of the liability of being told *"you didn't follow the law, you didn't enforce the law"* or they're afraid of a baby becoming blind and then being sued. So they have a lot of fear that makes them pressure women and families into getting the erythromycin ointment, and one of the ways that they will pressure women is to say *"well, if you decline, we have to report you to Child Protective Services"* and that's the worst case scenario of what you might encounter if you decide to decline.

Sarah: And what does that really mean? I know you don't work for Child Protective Services, but have you seen what usually happens in those cases?

Dr. Dekker: I haven't personally, but there is a doula that worked really hard to get the law changed in Washington State. She wrote an article for my blog one time about how she changed the law. She talked to Child Protective Services and to a whole bunch of different people and basically discovered that if it's reported, since this can't really harm the baby that it's not something they're really going to act on, other than they may be coming to visit you to see what's going on. But according to her, they can't really do anything about it, unless, there's something else going on, like your partner is abusing you, you're using drugs or something like that.

So it's possible that they could call Child Protective Services and if you have something else going on that's endangering your child, then that could become an issue, but for the most part, what she told me, is that these complaints go into a box in a dark closet where nobody ever looks at them.

It's really more of an issue of the hospital trying to cover their own butt and say, *"we did everything we could to try to enforce this family to have eye ointment."*

So if you're going to decline it in one of those situations, you have to understand that you should think about what are the benefits and risks of fighting the system, and I think most parents don't want to fight.

I think it really depends on how much you're willing to make waves for the decision that you think is right for your baby.

Sarah: Great point! That's why we're doing what we're doing and you're doing what you're doing ... to give parents the best evidence based information to help them make the right decision for your family. There's no one right way to give birth, but there is a right way for you. And the same thing applies to decisions after birth.

The decisions I make for my family might not be the decision that you make, and that's ok. Having the knowledge and research evidence to making your decision will give you so much more confidence as a mom, even long after birth is over. Advocating for your family also helps you get better healthcare for your family and find a provider you can trust as a team member.

Thanks so much Dr. Dekker for pointing us back to the evidence and helping us make sense of it all!

Supporting Evidence

Dr. Dekker thoroughly explains the research and evidence as it pertains to putting the eye gunk on our babies' eyes after birth. If you'd like to read more on the research, here is all the evidence that she talks about:

- Ali, Z., D. Khadije, et al. (2007). "Prophylaxis of ophthalmia neonatorum comparison of betadine, erythromycin and no prophylaxis." J Trop Pediatr 53(6): 388-392.

- Blatt, A. J., J. M. Lieberman, et al. (2012). "Chlamydial and gonococcal testing during pregnancy in the United States." Am J Obstet Gynecol 207(1): 55 e51-58.
- Centers for Disease Control (2012). Chlamydia – CDC Fact Sheet.
- Centers for Disease Control (2010). STD trends in the United States: 2010 national data for gonorrhea, chlamydia, and syphilis.
- Chen, J. Y. (1992). "Prophylaxis of ophthalmia neonatorum: comparison of silver nitrate, tetracycline, erythromycin and no prophylaxis." Pediatr Infect Dis J 11(12): 1026-1030.
- Darling, E. K. and H. McDonald (2010). "A meta-analysis of the efficacy of ocular prophylactic agents used for the prevention of gonococcal and chlamydial ophthalmia neonatorum." J Midwifery Womens Health 55(4): 319-327.
- Hammerschlag, M. R., J. W. Chandler, et al. (1980). "Erythromycin ointment for ocular prophylaxis of neonatal chlamydial infection." Journal of the American Medical Association 224(20): 2291-2293.
- Hammerschlag, M. R., C. Cummings, et al. (1989). "Efficacy of neonatal ocular prophylaxis for the prevention of chlamydial and gonococcal conjunctivitis." N Engl J Med 320(12): 769-772.

- Hedberg, K., Ristinen, T. L., Soler, J. T., et al. (1990). "Outbreak of erythromycin-resistant staphylococcal conjunctivitis in a newborn nursery." Pediatr Infcect Dis J 9(4): 268-273.
- Isenberg, S. J., L. Apt, et al. (1995). "A controlled trial of povidone-iodine as prophylaxis against ophthalmia neonatorum." N Engl J Med 332(9): 562-566.
- Lund, R. J., M. A. Kibel, et al. (1987). "Prophylaxis against gonococcal ophthalmia neonatorum. A prospective study." S Afr Med J 72(9): 620-622.
- Medves, J. M. (2002). "Three infant care interventions: reconsidering the evidence." J Obstet Gynecol Neonatal Nurs 31(5): 563-569.
- Schaller, U. C. and V. Klauss (2001). "Is Crede's prophylaxis for ophthalmia neonatorum still valid?" Bulletins of the World Health Organization 79(3): 262-263.
- Standler, R. B. (2006). Statutory law in the USA: requiring silver nitrate in eyes of newborns. Published online at http://www.rbs2.com/SilvNitr.pdf

In Short

Putting Erythromycin eye ointment in our babies' eyes is one of those things that doesn't really seem to be a big deal, at least from the outside. But for some mamas, it might be another "thing" that hospitals routinely do that's not based on medical evidence and can't be enjoyable for baby, which therefore makes it unnecessary.

It's definitely a good idea to find out if the erythromycin eye ointment is mandated in your state. If it's not, then this is a post-birth decision you'll want to talk over with your partner and make before labor.

If you'd like to opt out of your baby getting eye ointment, we encourage you find out what the laws are in your state. The best way to do this is to contact your state's health department.

As with most government websites, the health department sites that we went to were a disaster! We couldn't find any information about state laws and the eye ointment (or vitamin k which we talk about next). So talking to someone on the phone from your state's health department is probably the best way to go. If that doesn't work, ask your provider. Then sit down with your provider and have a good ole fashioned heart to heart. Consider getting screened for STDs. Compile all this information and make your decision.

***

Wow mama. We are cruising through all these ways to boost our baby's health after birth. While eye ointment isn't that thrilling of a topic to learn about, - we wanted to include it in this book about this super amazing time after you meet your baby. Once you hold your baby and look into their eyes (gooped or not), you'll never be the same again. It's amazing and something to get really, really excited for. Yeehaw!

Take Action

1.   Decide if this is something you want to do or opt out of doing.

2.   Get excited about having an adventure and call your health department! Find out what your state's laws are about the eye ointment and if there are any forms you need to fill out if you would like to opt out.

3.   If you don't get anywhere with the health department, call your hospital or birth center. Find out what they know about erythromycin eye ointment. They should have copies of any forms you might need to sign.

Chapter 8

How Vitamin K Can Save Your Baby After Birth. What's the Best Way to Give It?

with Dr. Robert Sidonio Jr., Pediatric Hematologist, Dad
Dr. Anna Morad, Director of Newborn Nursery,
Pediatrician, Mom

You know when we were little and we'd grab our neighborhood friends and have slumber parties, play "truth or dare" and that game "telephone?"

Remember those days?

Dang. Those were some good 'ole {carefree} days, weren't they?

Ok, so if you have no clue what I'm talkin' about, then let me fill you in. Me and all my homies would sit in a circle and one person would come up with a message like *"Allie has a ginormous crush on Brandon but played spin the bottle at the roller skating rink and kissed Kyle."*

Then the message would get repeated from person to person, in a whispering sort of way, until it came back to the originator of the message. The last person would finally say out loud what they heard. And it usually sounded something like *"Allie went to the zoo and decided she wanted a monkey, so she found one on craigslist and begged her daddy to buy it and bring it to the skating rink."*

Seriously. That's what happens. If you've played this little game, you totally know what I'm talking about, right?

And everyone laughs and it's hilarious.

So why in the heck am I bringing this up?

Because this game of telephone is often what happens when we "google" something birth related, read blogs, talk to friends who talked to friends who talked to whatshername ……. and then make real life decisions based on some mumbojumbo we heard 10 times removed. Our decision ends up being based on misinterpreted hearsay that has no basis.

Well guess what?

Vitamin k is the girl in the circle who started the story, but whose story gets all jacked up by the end.

But here's the thing …vitamin k is a story we have to get right.

And the reason we have to get it right is because vitamin k could save our baby's life. Vitamin k has saved many babies lives.

Two of our physician friends recently told us that they're hearing an increased number of moms talk about vitamin k with inaccurate, wrong and non-evidence based information. Dr. Sidonio even said … *"There's a lot of bad information* [going around] *and not much supporting information on the internet."*

Because of this, the same two physicians have seen an increased number of "vitamin k deficiency bleeding" cases in babies. These physicians believe those cases were preventable.

Had the mom (or couple) had accurate, evidence-based information, they believe the babies never would have had the problems that they did.

This chapter is here to stop the misinformation. And give you the accurate evidence based information you need to improve your precious little bundle's health!

We'll introduce you to these two doctors who will give you the evidence based facts on why giving your baby vitamin k at birth is so important for their health and how you can get it to protect your baby.

But first, here's the scoop.

In most hospitals, after birth, your baby will receive a vitamin k injection. This is part of the "standard of care" (code for: this is what we do...period.) that goes along with the eye ointment we talked about above.

And like we just mentioned, vitamin k is a super important.

It's important because vitamin k is thought to help prevent vitamin k deficiency bleeding. That's a fancy name for a blood disorder that prevents your baby's blood from clotting (which can cause internal bleeding and brain bleeding). The old term was called hemorrhagic disease of the newborn.

But what does the scientific evidence say about giving our babies vitamin k?

What does it even do? Is it necessary? If it's necessary, could we wait 2 months until their little bodies are more mature (beyond their first hour of life)? According to the evidence, is there a better way to give them vitamin k, while still getting all the protection and improved health?

These are great questions!

To lead us through vitamin k, we've found two of the country's top doctors at one of the leading hospitals in the country.

Dr. Robert Sidonio Jr. is a Pediatric Hematologist at Vanderbilt University's Hemostasis and Thrombosis Clinic (hematologists specialize in blood). And we also have Dr. Anna Morad, Assistant Professor of Pediatrics at Monroe Carrell Jr. Children's Hospital at Vanderbilt University and Director of Vanderbilt's Newborn Nursery.

Let's go, shall we?

***

"There are a lot of things in a newborn that aren't perfectly formed and fully functioning yet.

This is common.

It just takes a little time for everything in a new baby to be working and up to speed."

-Dr. Anna Morad

Sarah: What does vitamin K do for us? Why do we need vitamin k in our bodies?

Dr. Sidonio: When we're born there are certain coagulation factors and natural blood thinners that need vitamin k to activate them. When you're born, you actually have these all of the needed coagulation factors, but without vitamin k they're not activated so they can't do their job in clotting. And so that's why vitamin k's critical for newborns.

Sarah: Are you speaking English? Haha! So bring it down to my elementary level, what you're saying is that vitamin k helps your blood clot, correct?

Dr. Sidonio: That's right. Vitamin k activates your clotting factors so your blood clots normally.

Sarah: Babies are born with low vitamin k, why is that?

Dr. Sidonio: When babies are born, their bodies (gut) do not produce a particular kind of vitamin k that is needed to allow this clotting (There are two forms of vitamin k in our bodies. We get one from our diet and the other from our gut). So for that short period of time when their bodies aren't producing that one specific form of vitamin k, they have to rely on their diet of formula or breast milk to get all of their vitamin k.

Dr. Morad: And one thing I'd like to quickly add. Babies have a lot of things that are still developing when they are born. Their circulatory system isn't mature, that's why they have purple hands and feet. Their neurologic system isn't mature, that's why they have the primitive reflexes. [Primitive reflexes are the kicking, twitching and jerking that babies do.] Their liver doesn't work all that great, that's why they get jaundice.

So there are a lot of things in a newborn that aren't perfectly formed and fully functioning yet. This is common. It just takes a little time for everything in a new baby to get working and be up to speed.

Sarah: At what point do babies' vitamin k levels reach their normal level?

Dr. Sidonio: Usually the vitamin k deficiency intensifies in the first week, then most children seem to reach adequate vitamin k stores by one month of age and definitely by four to six months of age. We're most concerned about that first month because babies don't really have as much Vitamin k as they need. By four to six months, the levels are similar to what a full-grown adult would be.

Sarah: What happens if babies don't have adequate vitamin k levels?

Dr. Morad: Sometimes nothing. We have babies who don't get their vitamin k, for whatever reason, and they do just fine. But some babies with low levels of vitamin k will start bleeding, which is exactly what "vitamin k deficiency bleeding" is. If they were to bleed and their little bodies hadn't yet stored enough Vitamin k to clot the blood, which would stop the bleeding, that's a very serious problem. It's life threatening.

We don't fully know what causes the initial bleeding and why one baby would be at higher risk than another baby.

Sarah: Where might it happen or what's actually happening?

Dr. Sidonio: Some of the classic symptoms are: nosebleeds, I've seen that in a child during my training. Circumcision, if the circumcision is done at the time when there's vitamin k deficiency, you could see circumcision bleeding. We did have one child who had Gastro Intestinal (GI) bleeding or bleeding in the gut.

The good thing is that these are all "warning bleeding signs," meaning that once we saw the bleeding, we could do things to stop it and prevent it from becoming life threatening. Unfortunately, we have also seen some bleeding in the head, which didn't turn out as well.

Dr. Morad: Can I just say something Sarah?

We understand this is scary stuff to think about. We have kids too. It's not fun. But here's the thing, we're here to teach your moms how to prevent it from becoming a scary situation. As parents, we can't pretend this never happens and this isn't a risk for our babies.

But here's the great news! What we can do is make decisions that will minimize the risk as much as possible.

That's why we're here.

We're here to help you do that!

We're here teaching moms because we've seen an increased number of brain bleeds in babies. And this is very frustrating for us, especially as physicians, because we believe these were preventable.

And even more frustrating is that we've heard moms share with us some of the misinformation they've been told by their friends, and in some cases, even by birth educators (who were very "naturally minded").

We love the idea of making birth as natural as mom wants it to be. But we believe it's critically important, for baby's health, to make sure our information and our decisions are based on medical evidence.

Not hearsay.

We want to help your moms understand vitamin k and learn how they can take a few easy steps to prevent this from happening to their babies.

Sarah: I'm really glad you said that. This can definitely be scary to think about. But just like you said, our jobs are to look out for our baby's best interest. We don't need to dwell on this stuff, but having an understanding of it and knowing what the best

evidence based information will actually help us help our babies avoid it and stay healthy.

Ok, it makes sense to me that not being able to clot isn't a good thing. But am I right in that the main danger of having vitamin k deficiency is that it could result in bleeding in the brain?

Dr. Morad: Yes, the vessels in the brain are not particularly strong and so one of the things we worry about is that they'll bleed into their brain and we can't see it.

So those "warning bleeding signs" that Rob talked about, you can see. You can see when they bleed around their belly button. You can see when they're bleeding into their poop. But you can't see when they're bleeding into their brain and that is life threatening.

Unfortunately, babies can't really tell you when they first start to bleed, so a lot of times you don't know until they become lethargic, they don't respond to you, they can't eat, or maybe they have a seizure. So that's why we want to prevent this from happening in the first place.

Sarah: What is the history of giving vitamin k right after birth?

Dr. Morad: It's been a standard since 1961 in America.

Sarah: What led us to making it protocol in most, if not all, hospitals?

Dr. Sidonio: We've sort of known about this since the 1940s- that if we gave vitamin k we could prevent this bleeding. But it really took quite a long period of time and big policy changes until the American Academy of Pediatrics recommended it in 1961. And even after that point, it still took up to a decade for a lot of institutions and states to fully implement. In the 1960s, we recognized that if we intervened, we could pretty much eliminate this disorder, particularly when given through the intramuscular route. The goal is about reducing the risk of serious bleeding to near zero.

Sarah: Okay and we'll get more into that a little bit later. So what is the standard of care after babies are born, when do they receive the vitamin k injection?

Dr. Morad: Well every hospital probably does it a little differently.

We really want the baby to go immediately skin to skin with mom and so for the first hour, or at least until after completion of first feed, we don't really want any other interruptions.

We want for the baby to be skin to skin.

We do delay cord clamping for at least two minutes and then the baby's brought up to mom's chest for an hour or so, then afterwards we give the eye ointment and do the vitamin k injection. But you don't really want those things happening in the very first hour, you want it sort of at the end of that hour.

Sarah: What are the risks associated with giving them the vitamin k shot? I think this is where a lot of the misinformation kind of comes in. Can you clear this up for us?

Dr. Morad: Sure! Well, it's a shot, it hurts. It's best to do it while they're breastfeeding (or at least skin to skin), because that will help distract them from some of the discomfort. You can get a little redness at the site where it's given, just because it is a shot. It's important, in my opinion, to point out that the shot is the better form in which to give vitamin k to your baby. I know we're going to get into that later and there's a multitude of reasons for that.

We don't know of any confirmed risks for this particular vitamin. It's been used safely for a very long time.

Dr. Sidonio: I think people need to understand that this shot has been given to millions of children throughout the world. There are some places in some parts of the world where they prefer to use the oral route and we can talk about that later. The shot form is really the most effective way to pretty much eliminate this disorder. This is probably one of the safest injections that we have. It's very safe, it's been well tested, it's FDA approved. A lot of the risks are sort of theoretical from different parents.

Dr. Morad: Right, and a lot of the risks that get propagated on the internet, are risks that are associated with the IV infusion, not the intramuscular injection. So I think it's a really important point to say, that the delivery method by which your baby receives the vitamin k does make a difference. And then also the other thing is that there are certain brands of the vitamin k injection, which have been mentioned online, as being risky. That's not the type that we use. We actually use a preservative free form and so there are other forms of vitamin k out there. I would encourage parents to just ask.

Sarah: Can you clarify for us the difference between the intramuscular (injection) version and the IV version of the vitamin k?

Dr. Morad: That's a great question. When you look at the package insert, some of the risks that are listed on the packages pertain to the IV infusion, not the intramuscular injection.

Sarah: And why would that be? Is it just the way it's delivered into your baby's body?

Dr. Morad: It's just the delivery method. By getting the vitamin k through the IV infusion, you're putting something directly into the vein, even though the risk in the vein is quite low, specifically the anaphylaxis issue that you see reported. I don't know that those are risks for the intramuscular injection.

Dr. Sidonio: They're not. Anaphylaxis with the intramuscular form is very low.

Sarah: Normally when moms give birth, especially in a hospital setting, the vitamin k is going to be given to your baby in a shot form. It's not going to be an IV unless you have a sick baby.

Dr. Sidonio: That's right. The babies that receive the vitamin k through an IV are the infants in the intensive care setting during an illness of some sort.

Sarah: It's good to know that we can see the ingredients for each brand (to see various preservatives or no preservatives).

Dr. Morad: Exactly. The brand's package insert is going to list everything. They're required to list everything and so you really need to be aware of the actual risks for that particular brand's vitamin being given.

Sarah: Ok, let's jump to some of the "what people are saying" claims, because it really gets confusing. While I was preparing for this interview, I was thinking *"oh my gosh, no wonder why we're so confused, it's because there's a lot of conflicting information."* So let's go down the list.

Dr. Sidonio: There's a lot of bad information and not much information supportive of vitamin K on the internet. A long history of low rates of infants without life threatening bleeding should be testimony to how well it works.

Sarah: And I think the important thing is to go back to the research, the evidence, to see what the scientific proven evidence says. We're going to get to that in a minute. Let's go through some of the big objections that parents have had in the past about vitamin k. The first one I want to talk about is that the vitamin k injection gives babies 20,000 times their needed dose. Is this true and if so, is this a concern?

Dr. Sidonio: It does give a higher dose. The reason is that it's injected into the muscle and it's a fat soluble vitamin, so what that means, is that not all of that 20,000 times dose gets absorbed immediately. The dose allows the vitamin k to protect your baby over the next (and up to) 6 months. It prevents the vitamin K deficiency bleeding from happening, which can occur as late as 6 months from birth. So that's the reason why the dose is so high.

220

Sarah: Because I'm researching how I can help my baby most efficiently absorb the super beneficial vitamin k, let me ask you a questions ... on my bottle of vitamins, it says "for best absorption take one vitamin in the morning and then take another one in the evening." And since our bodies can only process so much at a time, isn't getting 20,000 times the amount of vitamin k my baby needs, and getting it all at once, isn't that a little extreme? Can a baby's body use all of that vitamin k, or is it just being wasted? Can you help us understand this?

Dr. Morad: It's just like any other long acting injection that you get. It sits there and gradually gets absorbed by their body.

Sarah: What I'm hearing you say is there's a difference in how your body processes getting a vitamin put directly into your muscle (via a shot) and swallowing the vitamin orally. Is that correct?

Dr. Sidonio: Yes. It's going to be processed differently. The problem with the oral version is that it doesn't protect you over a long period of time. And so the oral version you have to take multiple doses to provide the same protection, and even then it's still not as effective as the intramuscular version. This form is used in many European countries but the hospital support system is very different with home nurse visits and longer post pregnancy stays.

Sarah: One concern we've seen from some parents is that vitamin k shots have been linked to leukemia and cancer and autism. What evidence based information do you have about this?

Dr. Sidonio: The study[liv] that caused this concern came out in 1990 and a subsequent study came out 2 years later by the same group. Multiple studies thereafter combined older data and used better research methodology showing that there was absolutely no association (between leukemia and the vitamin k injection).

The problem is there are multiple articles that were published afterwards, which don't get put on the internet, and the one lingering article from 1990, that was debunked, remains on the internet.

Sarah: We mentioned before that not all vitamin k injections have the same ingredients in them. Your hospital uses a preservative free one. Other brands have preservatives in them. Can parents choose the brand that their baby receives? Is that possible?

Dr. Morad: That's an interesting question. I guess if parents researched it far enough ahead of time then they certainly could ask the hospital. There are preservative free brands. There are going to be additives because you have to keep it soluble, or in a liquid form. It's an important question to ask, but they would need to plan ahead for that because most hospitals have a contracted brand.

Sarah: Are there any other myths or reasons why, in your experience, parents have objected to the vitamin k injections?

Dr. Morad: Parents will sometimes say *"my baby was term"* or *"we're not going to circumcise"* or *"we will wait to circumcise for 8 days"* or *"my baby didn't have a traumatic birth, so they don't need it"*.

None of those are proven to protect our babies against vitamin K deficiency bleeding.

Dr. Sidonio: We've also seen girls with significant bleeding, so we know that it happens regardless of gender. The first week to the first month, that's when the highest risk of bleeding occurs.

Sarah: What is the likelihood that a baby will have vitamin k deficiency bleeding?

Dr. Sidonio: The most recent data has said there are about 6 cases per million births, assuming the shot has been given. If you don't give the shot, we may see up to 1 in 100 to 1 in 1000 babies get it. It depends on the situation.

The classic scenario is the exclusively breastfed baby, whose parents declined the vitamin k injection at birth. That's the classic scenario where it puts the child at the highest risk.

Sarah: And that's because breast milk doesn't have a lot of vitamin k, compared to formula. Right? Are there any other myths that you guys commonly hear that you think is important to talk about with our moms?

Dr. Sidonio: Anna you probably have seen this as well, but a lot of families feel that if the mother is able to eat a diet that's rich in vitamin k, that this injection will be unnecessary. Studies have been done and actually proven that you can't get the levels of vitamin k needed, that you can get with the injection. So we know that just changing your diet is not adequate to protect your baby.

Dr. Morad: There are families who believe if you delay the cord clamping that it will give your baby adequate vitamin k stores.

Both are not true.

Sarah: Those are two interesting thoughts and glad we clarified. Ok, let's move on now to other ways vitamin k can be given, without a shot right at birth.

Lets talk about orally, you guys mentioned a little bit about it. I found research that said the oral vitamin k was not as effective (or as quickly effective), but is a suitable option (instead of the injection). I know you mentioned earlier that you feel the shot is the better delivery method.

Dr. Morad: I don't think either of us would disagree with that. It's ok but it's not the best.

Dr. Sidonio: We look at the breakthrough cases [involving the oral vitamin k delivery method], particularly the ones that happened in

England, and they're always in the babies that never got that second or third dose of vitamin k.

So we have to rely on parents remembering to give their baby the multiple doses of oral vitamin k. When you give an intramuscular injection, you just give one dose one time and it's done, there's nothing else to do. We worry about parents remembering to give multiple doses of a vitamin k, that's not on a regular schedule, etc.

Dr. Morad: Ok and the other thing I would point out, if you've ever tried to give a baby an oral medication, think about the percentage that comes right back at you. A lot of times and depending on the baby, it's really difficult to get the full dose in orally.

That adds to the compliance issue, even if you're a parent and you're completely compulsive about giving it, it could still be a problem.

Sarah: This is a quote from the Cochrane Collaboration (an international committee of medical doctors of the highest caliber):

> *"Very similar rates of protection against classical and late hemorrhagic disease can be achieved by giving repeated oral doses, either 1 milligram weekly or 25 micrograms daily. Undertaking this form of oral prophylaxis requires that parents accept responsibility for ensuring the course is completed."*

Dr. Sidonio: That dosing regimen is quite difficult in which to comply and there are a couple of other alternative regimens that are more likely to be used...

In Japan and Switzerland, and I think in Germany too, they usually give 2 mg in the first couple of hours. And then they give another dose somewhere between day 3 and 10. Then they have to give another dose at about 1 month of age. You have to remember that people are in the hospital much longer in those countries after birth, so those first two doses can often be given before they're discharged. So they're only relying on one dose after one month of age. In America, most of us are out of the hospital with our children within 48 to 72 hours.

Sarah: Right, and for homebirth, you're never in the hospital and for birth center birth, you're there, maybe, for a few hours.

Dr. Sidonio: Another issue is that we also don't have an FDA approved oral version in the United States. They have a version that's approved in those countries, not available here.

Sarah: Do vitamins need to be FDA approved? What's the deal with that?

Dr. Morad: That's a great question. The vitamins that you're using for prophylaxis [that means for preventing a disease, etc.] for a known issue, it's best that they're FDA approved. But most vitamins do not fall under FDA approval.

Dr. Sidonio: You could pick up vitamins from a grocery store or from a vitamin store and they could lay claim that there's a milligram or two milligrams in there. But to be honest, if you analyzed it and there was less vitamin k in there than they said, there is absolutely nothing you could do about it because it's not regulated by the government. That falls under a different law.

Sarah: Ok I'm not going to beat a dead horse, but I kind of am, because I want to make sure we all understand this. I was reading Dr. Cees Vermeer's work on vitamin k, he's one of the leading experts who focuses on vitamin k. He says it doesn't matter if vitamin k is administered through injection of orally, as long as you're giving it to your baby, it will do the same job. What are your final thoughts on this?

Dr. Sidonio: Once it's in the bloodstream, it's going to work the same, so that's not the issue. The real question is how many infants that develop life-threatening bleeding are we willing to accept in this country? With the oral regimen, we are basically accepting a higher rate of vitamin K deficiency bleeding. I personally would love to make this disorder so rare that we can focus on other issues in infants.

Sarah: Let's say I'm a patient of yours at Vanderbilt and I decide that I don't want my baby to have a shot. Would it be possible for me to request my baby gets this orally instead?

Dr. Morad: We do not have that as part of our offering at this point in time, because it isn't FDA approved. What you're running up against is that we have an injectable vitamin that has no significant risk and it's proven to be incredibly effective. So why would we offer something that we know is not FDA approved and isn't as effective?

Now we do have families that opt for it and they will order it through other providers and give it independent of our system.

Sarah: Okay. Great info. It's important we know and understand all our options. Even with the best doctors on our team, the responsibility of being a parent rests on our shoulders. How long do babies need to supplement?

Dr. Sidonio: If they get the injection, that's it. Unless they have an underlying liver disorder or some gastrointestinal disorder, essentially there's no concern and there's no reason to follow up on it.

Sarah: And for those who are giving their babies oral vitamin k, it depends on the dosage obviously, but it would need to be several dosages over a period of several months, is that right?

Dr. Sidonio: Yes, if you use a very low dose. Your baby could be taking it as long as 13 to 14 weeks later, but that would have to be given daily and like I said you could utilize the three- dose version that I mentioned several of the other westernized countries are using.

Dr. Morad: Can I just say real quick? People assume that these parents who declined vitamin K did something wrong or they didn't have a good diet or that there was something wrong about the birth. And there's not.

These are smart, educated parents who have done their research. They're trying to make the best decisions, they're eating a good diet, they're breastfeeding. They're doing everything right.

That's the thing that's been most startling to me, the cases we've seen have not been predictable and people want to have a reason to predict it right? Everybody wants to look and say *"Oh... that's why."* These are mommies that would be your friends, they're normal families. So that's what I would like to get out there.

Dr. Sidonio: I would reiterate what Anna just said, these are well educated families. Most of them are college educated and spend a great amount of time researching. Unfortunately, some of them are relying too much on internet and hearsay, which can provide a lot of odd notions with no good data to back it up.

As you probably saw from that CDC report, the number of people that are declining vitamin k in the local Nashville area is over 25%. That's not particularly at Vanderbilt University, that's because of our effort largely by Anna, to really try to educate the families. But when you start to see up to 25% of the people declining it, we're going to see a lot of breakthrough cases unfortunately, something that we prefer not to see.

Sarah: Is there anything else you guys want to add?

Dr. Morad: Giving vitamin k is super cheap. It is a very inexpensive vitamin. Robert you know the cost on this, it is not expensive.

Dr. Sidonio: Less than a dollar. This is not something that the drug companies make money off of and at one point we were concerned that the companies would stop producing it or reduce the amount that they're making because it's not something lucrative for them. But we know, as a society, it's important for us to advocate for things like this.

Sarah: I'm really glad you mentioned that because that's one thing that's always in the back of my head now days, *"hmm... what are the economics here? Is the oral thing not done by a hospital because of a money issue?"* **So I'm really glad that you mentioned that.**

Dr. Sidonio: We don't make money off of a one-dollar injection. It's something that the hospital absorbs as part of standard care because it's such a small amount of money.

I also wanted to say that we are not against breastfeeding. We know that breast milk has 10x less vitamin k compared to formula. If the shot is given, then it's not a concern. We strongly support breastfeeding over formula feeding.

Dr. Morad: Oh yeah! Please clarify that, because we cannot say it enough, that we strongly encourage moms to breastfeed.

Sarah: Well a huge thank you to both of you for teaching us about vitamin k. And teaching us "the why," why it's so important to help our babies get it and how we can help them get it!

Supporting Evidence

Well Mama, if you decide to search for the research on vitamin k, you'll find an absolute ton! To be honest, it can be a bit overwhelming. So we've chosen a few of the best studies to share with you.

Does giving babies preventative (prophylaxis means the same thing as preventative) vitamin k work to reduce bleeding?

In 1992, a leading international pediatric journal (called Acta Paediatrica) published the findings of a study that was trying to figure out if the vitamin k (either through injection, IV, or oral) was effective in stopping hemorrhage in newborns. Here's what they found:

The effectiveness was 96.7% when vitamin k was given either through injection or IV and 80.4% for oral intake- the oral effectiveness was lower because the test only gave one oral dose.[lv] It has since been established that you need more than one oral dose for effective oral delivery of vitamin k.

According to studies done in Sweden and the USA, giving vitamin k through injection has pretty much eliminated vitamin k deficiency bleeding.[lvi]

There are plenty more where this came from and they all say the same thing. So I will spare you from repetition.

There is no dispute that vitamin k is effective in preventing vitamin k deficiency bleeding.

It works mamas.

Giving your baby vitamin k at birth improves their health through prevention.

Is the vitamin k injection (also called intramuscular) safe?

There was a review of research published in the Canadian Medical Association Journal (including six controlled trials that met the criteria of having a follow up 4 weeks after birth, at least 60 participants and a comparison of oral and intramuscular applications of the vitamin k) and they found that there was no compelling evidence that the vitamin k injection causes childhood leukemia or other cancer.[lvii]

In the next study, researchers looked at 420,000 babies who were given vitamin k through an injection. They found that there were no "significant complications" that happened as a result. They did bring up the fact that the psychological effect of injections on newborns (and mommies and daddies) are unknown. But concluded that the benefit of the vitamin k injection is greater than the potential psychological harm of having some pain from a shot.[lviii]

The American Association of Pediatrics wrote an article addressing the concerns about the vitamin k injection causing childhood leukemia and cancer. In analyzing the research, they found no relationship between the two.

Their conclusion was that the associated risks of babies having vitamin k deficiency bleeding (and even possibly dying because of it) far outweighed the small possibility that some day, that same baby could get cancer (which can't be scientifically linked to vitamin k injection in the first place).[lix]

But do we have to use an injection? What about the oral doses of vitamin k? Do they work & are they a good alternative?

An extensive review of all the studies was done spanning a 70-year period. Researchers were looking at the effectiveness of the oral dose of vitamin k compared to the injection.

They found oral dosing of vitamin k to be acceptable. But no one has come out and specifically said "hey, this is the dose and the type of (FDA approved) oral vitamin k you need to use." Once they do that, and everyone is on the same page (getting on the same page is called "protocol" in medical terminology) it could be routinely used in the U.S. [lx]

We can't stress enough, TALK TO YOUR PROVIDER. **We are presenting research, not telling you what doses to give or what to do.** It's incredibly important that you ask your doctor about oral vitamin k and what doses to give, if you choose to go that route.

Dr. Anton H. Sutor, a leading scientist in pediatric hemostasis (process which causes bleeding to stop) published a ton of research and articles about vitamin k. In one of them, he wrote, *"The major disadvantage of oral prophylaxis, namely, its lesser reliability in terms of intake and absorption, could be largely overcome by repeated administration."*[lxi]

The last research study I'll mention is a review done which looked at 11 randomized trials. They compared the injection to the oral or doing nothing at all. What they found was that both the injection and the oral dose improved coagulation at 1 to 7 days after birth. (That was for a single dose).[lxii]

According to the research studies, Oral doses are found to be completely acceptable in increasing babies' vitamin k levels when administered with the right dose and multiple times.

In Short

Shew! That was some intense research! Believe me when I say that digging into all that research made my head hurt, in good way of course.

So what did we learn from this chapter?

We learned that if you breastfeed, which is arguably the best for baby, your baby will be deficient in vitamin k until about six months of age. Research clearly shows that supplementing with vitamin k, either through injection or orally, helps to prevent vitamin k deficiency bleeding. This type of bleeding is incredibly serious and a potentially life threatening blood disorder.

The biggest drawback for doing the oral route, according to doctors and research, is that parents may forget to give their sweet bambinos this really important vitamin.

There are basically three types of vitamin k deficiency bleeding: early, classic and late.

Early bleeding happens within the first 24 hours after birth. This is rare. Classical bleeding happens anywhere from 24 hours after birth to one week. Signs include bleeding around the umbilical cord area, where your baby was circumcised, skin, nose, even blood in their poop and may mean internal bleeding in the brain. This happens in about .01% to 1.5% of newborns. Late bleeding is 2 to 12 weeks but can happen up to 6 months old. Babies who have late bleeding commonly will have brain bleeds. This happens in about 4-10 per 100,000 births.[lxiii]

Myth: Newborn levels of vitamin k return to "normal" on day 7. So there's no point in messing with supplementing vitamin k.

Fact: It can take up to 6 months for vitamin k levels to reach their ideal levels[lxiv]. The first month to two months are when your baby is at the greatest risk for having vitamin k deficiency bleeding- which is a fancy name for a blood disorder that prevents their blood from clotting and can cause internal bleeding including brain bleeds.

Myth: If my baby has a brain bleed, it's no big deal.

Fact: Brain bleeds vary in their seriousness but it's super, duper important to know that they are irreversible. Once your baby has a brain bleed, there is nothing that can be done to fix that brain bleed. Vitamin k can be given to your baby through an IV or injection, which will prevent further brain bleeds from happening.

Studies show that brain bleeds can mean developmental delays for your baby, or even cerebral palsy in some cases and in the worst cases, death. This stuff is no joke.

Myth: The injections can cause leukemia and other cancers.

Fact: The doctors who made this link between leukemia, cancers and the vitamin k injection based their claims off of a study done in Great Britain in 1970. The doctors saw a relationship between babies who had received the vitamin k and then later were diagnosed with leukemia or other cancers and concluded that babies who received the vitamin k injection doubled the incidence of childhood leukemia in kiddos 10 years and younger.[lxv] Remember how Dr. Sidonio mentioned that the American Academy of Pediatrics recommended all babies get vitamin k after birth in 1961? There has been no sharp increase in childhood leukemia since then[lxvi]. This myth has been debunked by the crap ton of research that has happened since then and no other researchers have found connections between the injection and leukemia or other cancers.

Myth: The oral form of vitamin k is not as effective as the injection.

Fact: The oral form of vitamin k is effective, it just may not work as quickly and requires multiple doses.[lxvii] As Dr. Sidonio pointed out, once the vitamin k gets into the body, its effectiveness is the same, whether it's an injection, oral or IV. The difference is the amount and how it goes into the body. As Dr. Morad pointed out, it can be tricky to give newborns oral vitamins, sometimes they spit up or the entire dose doesn't make its way into their mouths etc. So you may not know exactly how much your baby has actually received. This can be tricky, but not impossible, and is definitely something to think about as you consider your options.

It can be really easy to get stuck in all the details of vitamin k and forget that vitamin k is not bad, it's a vitamin and a very needed part of our bodies that helps our blood to clot. Vitamin k also helps prevent the hardening of the arteries, so it keeps your heart healthy, it helps build healthy bones and can even help prevent cancer. Sometimes vitamin k is called "the forgotten vitamin" because it does so many great things for our bodies that are overlooked. Poor thing.

Some of you may not have much of a choice when it comes to whether or not you'll have your baby get vitamin k- in some states its law- just like with the eye ointment. But, you may still have some options. For example, you can ask to do the oral administration of vitamin k.

As Dr. Morad mentioned, in the US, there is no oral vitamin k that has been approved by the FDA. I wasn't aware that the FDA needed to approve vitamins, but Dr. Morad said that for preventive reasons (prophylaxis use) the FDA weighs in. But there are over the counter vitamin k supplements that can be purchased. **It's important to talk to your doctor about this whole subject, no matter what you decide to do**.

Find out if oral is available to you in the hospital and if not, you will need to decide if you want to administer it at home yourself. I'm guessing that if giving your baby vitamin k is important to you, you'll set a reminder in your phone and get 'er done.

"Forgetful parents" is the beef most researchers had with this method ..."*will the parents remember to give their babies this super, crazy important vitamin supplement?*" Thank God for smart phones, calendars, spouses and family members who you've charged with calling you EVERY time you need to give your 'lil cutie pie that vitamin k, thereby making sure you can't possibly forget.

We're not advocating for oral, it's your choice. We're just pointing out that if giving vitamin k was super important to you to help prevent your baby from having any bleeding, we believe you'd a way to make 100% darn certain you couldn't possibly forget.

If you're still thinking you want to do "one and done" with the injection, know that not all injections are created equal.

Just like a fruit smoothie kind of drink at the store, some have better things inside than others. Some you don't want.

READ THE PACKET INSERT that manufacturers of these injections must include with them.

How do you do this? During your hospital tour, ask for one:

"Hi, we'll be giving birth here soon and would like to know, what brand of vitamin k injections do you use? We'd like to see one of the package inserts. Thanks so much!"

If you need help reading the packet insert, grab a nurse and have them give you a 5 minute tutorial, before you leave the hospital (from your tour). Write down your notes, and better yet, bust out your smartphone and take a pic of the packet insert. Then Google it and see what all those long ingredient names actually are and then at your next appointment, go over all this with your awesome provider.

Dr. Morad mentioned that the brand they use at Vanderbilt contains no preservatives, so we know it is possible for hospitals to use brands that have fewer ingredients but still do the job.

This is a huge distinction mamas. **This is really important.**

You may be wondering *"well what happens if the hospital uses one of the yucky, preservative filled vitamin k shots?"* Great question.

Talk to your provider and find out what your options are. Remember how you and your doctor or midwife are the dream team? This is a perfect example of working together to find a solution. The hospital might be able to order you another brand, or your doctor can get it for you, or you can get it from the health department yourself.

Where there's a will, there's a way.

No one will look out for your baby like you. If you've decided on doing a vitamin k injection, great! Make sure it's a good one. Not just any old one. Your baby is worth it!

Whenever I'm mulling through a goldmine of evidence based info like this, in order not to get overwhelmed, I sort of dial it down and ask myself a simple question... is it worth it?

Even though it might feel a little uncomfortable asking the hospital or my doctor a few questions about vitamin k ... Is it worth gambling that my baby might be the 1 in 1,000 who has vitamin k deficiency bleeding?

That is a question that you and only you can answer.

It may be a no brainer, or it could be something you really need to think about or even research more on your own (we've given you lots and lots of links to make it easier for you).

The point is, no one should make this decision for you, it should be yours, because your baby is yours. And no one is more concerned or responsible for your baby's health than you.

Way to go mama, so many mamas don't even know how easily they can improve their baby's health right after birth. Big kudos to you for investing some time to help your baby do a ton of miracles after birth! They will show their appreciation to you by some big blowouts, spit ups and sleepless nights. They love you mama. They do.

Take Action

1. Have a sit down with your significant other and re-read this chapter. Then decide if you will be:
    - ☐ Getting the vitamin k injection
    - ☐ Doing the oral vitamin k with appropriate, multiple, oral doses
    - ☐ Declining the vitamin k in both forms

2. Talk to your provider about your decision.
3. Write it in your birth plan to keep everyone informed.

Where do I go from here?

Whew doggies.

First of all ... congrats! You're investing in your baby's health and future ... there's no better investment.

Maybe your first next step should be to take a nap. Cause honestly, when is that ever a bad idea? Or you might be hungry, so grab a snack. Whatever you decide to do, celebrate your dedication to the cuteness you'll soon meet!

There is a lot of information to chew on in here. This is the time when I like to remind our readers about a motto we have at Your Baby Booty: *"There's no one right way to birth a baby, but there's a right way for you."* This is where I don't tell you what to do next because that is only something that you can do. Only you and your partner can figure out what is best for you and your baby. Next steps for you may mean that you take a nice warm bath and bask in the flow of hormones coursing through your body. Or that you have a heart to heart with your provider and let them know everything that you've been learning and make sure you are all on the same page.

It could mean you print some of the templates and downloads we've provided and have a chat with your spouse (and maybe even ask them to read this book) and write your birth plan together.

But do something.

Small actions give you BIG results. Even just a little tiny action that takes you one small step closer towards your goal builds momentum. Then comes confidence. It snowballs.

Congrats!! ...Awesome job! You're almost done reading this book ...

Take 1 minute...

Grab your journal. Take 1 minute and write down the ONE most important thing you learned from this book and the ONE thing you want to do after reading this book. Make a check mark box next to it. When you're done doing that one thing, cross it off your list. Ahhhh. Doesn't that feel good?

Final thoughts on the next page ...

Final thoughts...

Hi mama! We loved writing this book for you. There was <u>a lot</u> to research, but it's all such important info!

What if ...

... your birth class or your provider just came out and said ... *"Ok, here's how we can improve your baby's health, BIG TIME, in the first hour after they're born. Let's walk through all your options and look at the research evidence so you can understand the opportunity you have to help give them a BIG health boost that'll last them their entire lives."*

Since we've never heard of that happening, we wanted to write the book that would do it for you.

Isn't it amazing how much we can help our sweet little baby's health?!? And how easily we can help? And geez, shouldn't every mom be taught these things?

Wherever you are in your journey, remember there are millions of women who have gone before you who had apprehensions just like you (*ahemmm ... I'm one of them*), and have done it. It's normal. It's okay.

You can do it, too. You can!

You were made to do this, wherever and however you choose. It's pretty cool that we women with children share a common bond of perseverance, of strength, of digging deep and seeing parts of ourselves we never thought we'd see.

The journey to the MotherLand is one amazing ride. Challenging for sure. But well worth every second when you meet your baby and fall in love.

Just remember… even when you feel like you can't…you can do it. **You are doing it!**

Our love to ya,

Sarah & Steve Blight

Can we ask a favor? *If you liked the book, it'd mean the world to us if you'd use 2 minutes to write a quick Amazon review sharing how this book helped you. We've worked hard to bring you a book that would impact your pregnancy & birth - your review would really help Birth Book reach more moms during pregnancy and birth. It's super easy and fast to do (literally takes just a few minutes)…*

1. *Go to Amazon.com and type in "Birth Book #2) then click on the gold Birth Book #2 title.*
2. *Click "Customer Reviews"(it's below the title, next to the stars & in-between the parenthesis)*
3. *Click on the "Create your own review" button (on the left side).That's it!*

Thank you so much, we're very grateful! ☺

If you liked this book... check out

Birth Book #1: How to Be Fearless in Birth, Find the Best Doctor or Midwife, Have Less Pain in Labor.

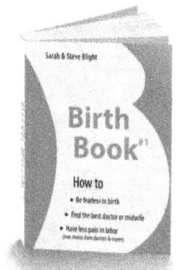

Birth Book #1 is full of true stories, candid conversations, important insights, and tips from top doctors and moms. They open up, get real and share with you what 100s of moms and over 70 combined years of "giving birth" experience has taught them about childbirth. Their knowledge becomes yours, so you can have an easier labor & healthy birth with your baby!

You'll also see the best research & medical evidence on giving birth. A lot of pregnancy books talk *about* "giving birth." *Birth Book* actually shows you *"how to have* a healthy birth" and gives you the evidence to back it up.

S. Elsben said *"I read this book while pregnant and loved it. It was soothing to read and full of helpful insights from other moms. I used several of the tips mentioned during labor and they helped me stay calm and confident. I had a beautiful birth experience, partly because of my midwives team within the hospital and partly because this book gave me permission to have a wonderful experience."*

Patty was pretty fired up and said, *"Yes, yes, yes! This is a short book but long on information. It is easy to read and can help new moms explore their feelings about what might be their best birthing experience. Thank you for a great birth book!"*

AVAILABLE ON AMAZON.COM

Going to the MotherLand: things to know for your journey.

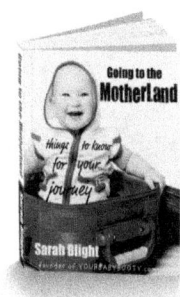

Sarah's debut book Going to the MotherLand is the honest-to-goodness, uncensored scoop about a first-time mama's journey through conception, raging hormones, pregnancy woes, getting baby out and figuring out what the hell to do next. Written for real moms with real questions, reading this book feels more like you're chatting it up with your best friend (with favorite beverage in hand) than reading a "pregnancy and childbirth book."

Carrie said *"Such a great read for anyone planning a journey to the new and strange land of parenting. It's filled with hilarious commentary, combined with honest and well-researched dialogue about pregnancy, birth, and the postpartum period. I wish this book had been on my shelf for babies #1 and #2. Maybe it'll inspire me to try for #3!"*

Natalie said *"Every mom should read this book! She had me laughing throughout! Easy to read and educational! Highly recommended to many friends already!"*

AVAILABLE ON AMAZON.COM

**Want to know when our next book is released? Just drop your email here:

http://book.yourbabybooty.com/future-books/

Or just say hi, I'd love to hear from you! Email me at Sarah@yourbabybooty.com

Thank You

Walking along your journey to the motherland can be lonely, tiring, super exciting, fun, frustrating, and at times, monotonous (hello mountain of laundry...didn't we just have a rendez-vous?) You're tirelessly devoted to your pregnancy, your baby, yourselves, and your families. Thank you for sharing this sweet part of your journey with us.

A super special thanks to Dr. Buckley, Dr. Jain, Mavis Schorn, Barbara Harper, Dr. Sidonio, Dr. Morad, and Dr. Dekker! Learning from you all is a huge privilege. Thanks for sharing your knowledge and experience with all of us.

Thanks also to all the mamas who gave us feedback on this book to make it rock solid during the editing portion of this process. We appreciate it like crazy.

One Last Thing...

If you believe your friends would get something valuable from Birth Book, please review our book on Amazon and GoodReads or share with your fellow preggos on Facebook. Your sharing will help us reach our goal of helping 100,000 moms!

Downloads & Extras

The next few pages contain hard copies of the links that we've created for you with Summaries of Evidence and Questions for you to ask your provider. Enjoy!

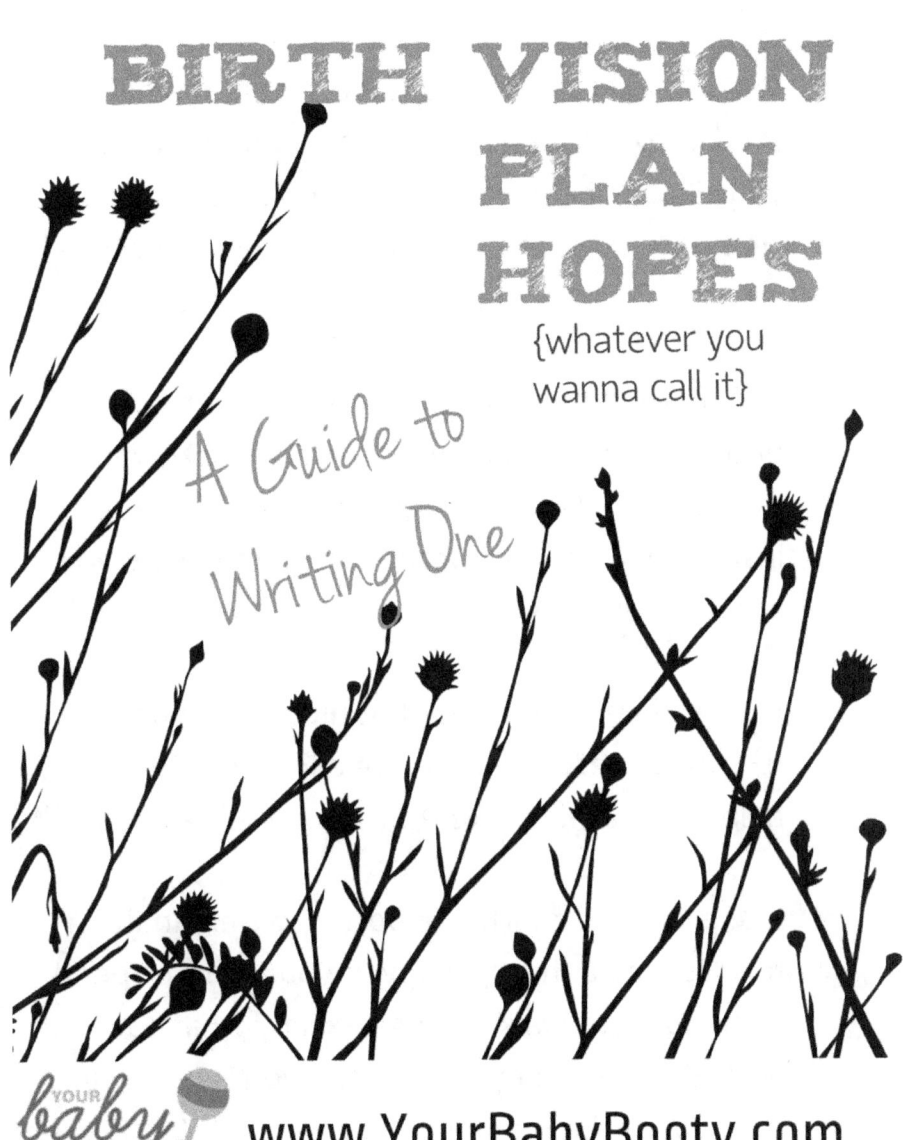

BIRTH VISION PLAN HOPES

{whatever you wanna call it}

A Guide to Writing One

YOUR baby BOOTY   www.YourBabyBooty.com

My Birth Vision Guide
Helpful Tips to Get You Started

✓ Use this guide as it's intended, a guide to help you *think through* items you might want to include in your Birth Vision- your Birth Desires- your Birth Hopes- your Birth Plan (whatever you want to call it!)

✓ You may want to copy and paste sections of this, or use this as a jumping off point to make your own Birth Vision in paragraphs or sentences instead of a checklist format, or if you want, you can use this, as is.

✓ Be specific and use clear but nice, kind wording (the nurses especially will be a lot more friendly & helpful if they feel like they're not being attacked).

✓ Make sure your birth support, spouse, family, friends, doula, have a copy of your Vision. Spend 15 minutes to walk through exactly what you want & ensure they understand your wishes. In the heat of the moment you'll be more focused on working through contractions than what you hope for your baby's birth to be (that's why support, who are on the same page, is CLUTCH!). Those 15 minutes spent might mean the difference between you smoothly accomplishing your plan...or getting something you didn't want.

✓ Remember to hold this vision loosely. Births often don't go as we think they will, remain flexible in your approach & keep the end goal in sight. When you have a plan, you're actually better prepared to handle changes because you've thought through your options. Woohoo! Get Excited!

My Birth Vision Guide

Birth Support
I'd like to have the following people with me in the labor/delivery room...

Room Ambiance
I would like:
- ☐ To bring my own music
- ☐ Use my own essential oils
- ☐ To take my own video/photos

Hospital Admittance
If I'm not in active labor, I'd like to go home.
Once I'm admitted, I'd like:
- ☐ my partner to be allowed to stay with me at all times
- ☐ only my practitioner, nurse, and guests to be present (i.e., no residents, medical students, or other hospital personnel)
- ☐ to wear my contact lenses, as long as I don't need a c-section
- ☐ to eat if I wish to
- ☐ to try to stay hydrated by drinking clear fluids instead of having an IV
- ☐ to have a heparin or saline lock
- ☐ to walk and move around as I choose

Labor
I would like to:
- ☐ be allowed to progress in labor without feeling rushed and would like to have my labor augmented only if absolutely necessary
- ☐ use a birthing stool
- ☐ use a birthing chair
- ☐ use a squatting bar

- [ ] use a birthing pool/tub

I'd like to bring the following with me:
- [ ] birthing stool
- [ ] beanbag chair
- [ ] birthing pool/tub
- [ ] birth ball
- [ ] other:

_____

Monitoring

As long as the baby and I are doing fine, I'd like to:
- [ ] have intermittent electronic fetal monitoring
- [ ] have continuous monitoring

Induction

- [ ] I do not want to be induced unless medical evidence supports it (ie baby or I are in danger).

If induction becomes necessary, I would like to:
- [ ] Discuss all the options with the doctor or midwife prior to starting
- [ ] Have my membranes stripped
- [ ] Have my water broken
- [ ] Use herbs
- [ ] Use prostaglandin
- [ ] Use Pitocin

Pain Medication

I'd like to try the following:
- [ ] acupressure
- [ ] counter-pressure
- [ ] bath/shower
- [ ] breathing techniques
- [ ] visualization
- [ ] self-talk
- [ ] hot/cold therapy
- [ ] self-hypnosis

- [ ] massage
- [ ] medication
- [ ] other:

_____

- [ ] Please don't offer me pain medication. I'll request it if I need it.

If I decide I want medicinal pain relief, I'd prefer:
- [ ] regional analgesia (an epidural and/or spinal block)
- [ ] narcotics
- [ ] nitrous oxide (laughing gas)

Perineum

I have been doing perineal massage, squats and kegels to prepare for birth, please protect my perineum by:
- [ ] Doing massage
- [ ] Using oil

I would rather:
- [ ] Have an episiotomy
- [ ] Tear naturally

Delivery

When it's time to push, I'd like:
- [ ] To do so when I feel like I need to (instinctive)
- [ ] Coach me on when to push and for how long

I'd like to try different positions for pushing like:
- [ ] semi-reclining
- [ ] side-lying position
- [ ] squatting
- [ ] hands and knees
- [ ] whatever feels good to me at that moment

During delivery, I'd like:

- [ ] to use a mirror (see what's going on)
- [ ] to touch my baby's head as he/she crowns
- [ ] absolute quiet
- [ ] my partner to help "catch" our baby

Immediately After Delivery

I'd like:

- [ ] to hold my baby right away - any procedures that aren't urgent can wait including measurements.
- [ ] do skin to skin for 1 hour, uninterrupted
- [ ] to breastfeed as soon as possible
- [ ] **not** to get Pitocin after I deliver the placenta unless it's necessary
- [ ] to wait until the umbilical cord stops pulsating before it's clamped and cut (delayed cord clamping)
- [ ] my partner to cut the umbilical cord

Cord Blood Banking

We're planning to:

- [ ] donate cord blood to a public bank
- [ ] bank cord blood privately
- [ ] neither

Postpartum

After delivery, I'd like:

- [ ] all newborn procedures to take place in my presence
- [ ] my partner to be with the baby at all times if I can't be there
- [ ] to stay in a private room
- [ ] to have a cot provided for my partner
- [ ] 24-hour rooming-in with my baby
- [ ] my baby to room-in with me only when I'm awake
- [ ] my baby brought to me for feedings only
- [ ] to make my decision later depending on how I'm feeling
- [ ] my other children brought in

Newborn Procedures
We **would like** the following for our baby:
- ☐ Eye ointment
- ☐ Vitamin K injection
- ☐ Vitamin K oral
- ☐ Hepatitis B vaccine
- ☐ Our baby bathed
- ☐ Blood sugar testing

We are choosing **NOT to have** the following for our baby:
- ☐ Eye ointment
- ☐ Vitamin K injection
- ☐ Vitamin K oral
- ☐ Hepatitis B vaccine
- ☐ Our baby bathed
- ☐ Blood sugar testing

Circumcision
We have decided:
- ☐ Not to circumcise our son
- ☐ To circumcise our son
- ☐ One or both of us would like to be present

Breastfeeding
- ☐ I would like to see a lactation consultant before going home.

I will be:
- ☐ Exclusively breastfeeding
- ☐ Giving my baby formula
- ☐ Combining formula and breast milk

I do not want:
- ☐ Glucose water or pacifiers given to my baby
- ☐ Formula given to my baby

Cesarean Section

If I have a c-section, I'd like:

- [ ] my partner in the operating room at all times
- [ ] our doula to be in the operating room
- [ ] to be as alert as possible, please don't give me drugs which will knock me out
- [ ] the screen lowered a bit so I can see my baby being delivered
- [ ] soft music playing
- [ ] Dr to deliver baby slowly and gently to mimic vaginal birth (if possible)
- [ ] our baby given to my partner (if possible)
- [ ] the baby held up to my face so I can see him/her
- [ ] baby placed on my chest to do skin to skin with assistance from birth support immediately after delivery
- [ ] spouse to do skin to skin with baby if it's not possible for me to do skin to skin immediately after delivery
- [ ] a nurse to take photos of my partner and I with the baby
- [ ] to breastfeed my baby as soon as possible

Additional Thoughts:

HOW TO ASK FOR
SKIN TO SKIN:

"Do you promote and encourage skin to skin immediately after baby is born?"

If they say "no" then you ask:

"Are you familiar with the leading research and evidence that supports it?"

If they say "yes", then you say:

"So you're familiar with Dr. Edgar Rey and Dr. Hector Martinez who discovered the incredible benefits of Kangaroo Care (skin to skin) in Bogota Columbia and saw their mortality rate drop 80%"
–then you show them the summary of evidence (below) and hand it to them.

Then you say:

"My husband and I would love to have an increased success in breastfeeding, less anxiety, better bonding. We would love for our baby to have an easier time transitioning outside the womb, have easier time with respiratory adjustments, regulation of body temperature and getting their heart rate into a settled rhythm just like the best research and evidence shows. We would love to spend the first two hours getting to know each other and would like for you guys to wait to measure, weigh and assess baby until after we're done, or do it while baby is on me."

If they object, or say that their nurses have protocol or timelines they need to accomplish things in you say:

"I'm sure that you as my provider, and nurses also, as well as the hospital would love for us to walk away from our birth experience satisfied and recommending your services and the hospital to our friends and family. Nothing will make us happier then being able to spend this important "golden hour" after birth with just our immediate family. That's one of the reasons we hired you, because we trusted that you would work with us to ensure that our birth is accomplished with evidence based practices. So how do we make this happen?"

If they still object, then schedule a visit with the hospital administrative staff, who oversee customer satisfaction (you ARE a customer after all).

Simply go over the evidence, hand them the summary of evidence and go through it with them

SUMMARY OF EVIDENCE
Skin to Skin

Moore, E. R., G. C. Anderson, et al. (2012). "Early skin-to-skin contact for mothers and their healthy newborn infants." Cochrane Database Syst Rev 5: CD003519.

> **The study:** A review of 34 randomized controlled trials including 2,177 mother-newborn pairs.
>
> **Result:** Positive effect of early skin to skin care on breastfeeding at one to four months post birth. Skin to skin enhanced the duration of breastfeeding. Late preterm infants had better cardio-respiratory stability with early skin to skin care. Blood glucose 75 to 90 minutes after birth was significantly higher in skin to skin care babies.

Affonso D, et al. Reconciliation and healing for mothers through skin-to-skin contact provided in an American tertiary level intensive care nursery. Neonatal Network, 1999,12:25-32

> **The study:** The Neonatal Network published a book highlighting various ways that mothers and preterm babies can benefit from skin to skin.
>
> **Result:** One major finding was that mothers who do skin to skin say they are less stressed when doing skin to skin as opposed to receiving the conventional hospital care. And they also say that they have more confidence, self-esteem and are more fulfilled.

Bystrova K, ET AL. Early Contact Versus Separation: Effects on Mother-Infant Interaction One Year Later. Birth, 2009 Jun:36(s):97-109.

The Study: Researchers looked at 176 mama, baby pairs. These pairs were split into four groups. In the first group, babies did skin to skin with their mamas after birth and then "roomed in" with them in the hospital. In the second group, the babies were dressed, their mamas held them and they roomed in with them. In the third group, the babies were kept in the nursery after birth and the entire time their mama was in the hospital. In the fourth group, the babies were kept in the nursery after birth but roomed in with their mamas during their hospital stay.

Result: Results showed that 1 year later, the skin to skin contact or early suckling or both when compared to separation, positively affected the infants' sensitivity to their mama. It also positively affected their self-regulation and how they reciprocated towards their mama.

World Health Organization (2003). Kangaroo mother care: A practical guide. Geneva, World Health Organization, Department of Reproductive Health and Research.

The guide can be found here:

http://whqlibdoc.who.int/publications/2003/9241590351.pdf

The Study: 47 healthy mother-baby pairs were randomized to receive kangaroo care (skin to skin) shortly after birth or standard care (no kangaroo care). The kangaroo care group started skin to skin 15 minutes after birth and did skin to skin for one hour.

Ferber s., I. Makhoul. The Effect of Skin-to-Skin Contact (Kangaroo Care) Shortly After Birth on the Neurobehavioral Responses of the Term Newborn: A Randomized, Controlled Trial. <u>Pediatrics</u>, 2003, DEC.

> **Result:** Kangaroo care seems to influence state organization, and "motor system modulation" of the newborn after birth.

IN BRIEF

This is a tiny sampling of the best medical research and evidence supporting skin to skin (kangaroo care).

Mothers and babies enjoy lifelong benefits from skin to skin including:

1. Earlier breastfeeding, which leads to higher rates of success and longer duration.
2. Heart rate, respiration and body temperature more likely to be stable.
3. Less crying.
4. Beneficial increase in blood sugar.
5. Helps baby's motor system adjust.
6. Less anxiety for mom.
7. Less breast engorgement/pain 3 days after birth.

HOW TO ASK FOR
skin to skin after C-section:

1. Ask for it at your prenatal appointment, or if it's an emergency C-section, ask for it beforehand. Say something like this:

"Do you promote and encourage skin to skin immediately after baby is born?"

or

"It's really important to my husband and I that I can do skin to skin with our baby immediately after birth as long as baby and I are doing well."

If they say "no" then you ask:

"Are you familiar with the leading research and evidence that supports it?"

If they don't seem to be, point them to the Summary of Evidence on the next page.

2. If they push back and say they don't do it, protocol, etc, then ask them if you could try it one time, print them a copy of the 11 steps to doing skin to skin after c-section, (below). And show that you're willing to lead them through it because you're educated about this, confident and super prepared. You're ready!

SUMMARY OF EVIDENCE
Skin to Skin After C-Section

Gouchon, S., D. Gregori, et al. (2010). "Skin-to-skin contact after cesarean delivery: an experimental study." <u>Nurs Res</u> 59(2): 78-84.

> **The study**: 34 pairs of mothers and newborns born by elective c-section were randomized to skin to skin care or routine care. Temporal artery temperatures were taken at 30 minute intervals.
>
> **Result:** Babies who did skin to skin after c-section were not at risk for hypothermia. Mean temperatures were almost identical in the two groups after 30 minutes and 120 minutes. The skin to skin babies attached to the breast earlier than the other group and were breastfed exclusively or prevalently at discharge and following at 3 months. Mothers in the skin to skin group expressed high levels of satisfaction with the skin to skin "intervention."

Moore, E. R., G. C. Anderson, et al. (2012). "Early skin-to-skin contact for mothers and their healthy newborn infants." <u>Cochrane Database Syst Rev</u> 5: CD003519.

> **The study:** A review of 34 randomized controlled trials including 2,177 mother-newborn pairs.
>
> **Result:** Positive effect of early skin to skin care on breastfeeding at one to four months post birth. Skin to skin enhanced the duration of breastfeeding. Late preterm infants had better cardio-respiratory stability with early skin to skin care. Blood glucose 75 to 90 minutes

after birth was significantly higher in skin to skin care babies.

Nolan, A. and C. Lawrence (2009). "A pilot study of a nursing intervention protocol to minimize maternal-infant separation after Cesarean birth." J Obstet Gynecol Neonatal Nurs 38(4): 430-442.

The study: 50 women having live, term, singleton, repeat c-section were randomized. A nursing protocol was created and administered which minimized the amount of spatial, tactile, olfactory, auditory and visual separation post c-section.

Result: Babies that had less separation had earlier first contact and feedings, a longer period before first bath. Differences were found in the intervention and control groups in respiratory rates and infant temperatures.

Smith J, Plaat F, Fisk N. The natural caesarean: a woman-centred technique. BJOG 2008;115:1037–1042

This article describes exactly how to go about keeping a sterile environment in the OR while enhancing mother, baby bonding which leads to increased rate and duration of breastfeeding, reduces infant crying and increases maternal affection and bonding.

World Health Organization (2003). Kangaroo mother care: A practical guide. Geneva, World Health Organization, Department of Reproductive Health and Research.

The guide can be found here:

http://whqlibdoc.who.int/publications/2003/9241590351.pdf

Velandia, M., K. Uvnas-Moberg, et al. (2012). "Sex differences in newborn interaction with mother or father during skin-to-skin contact after Caesarean section." Acta Paediatr 101(4): 360-367.

The study: 37 healthy babies were randomized to receive 25 minutes of skin to skin with either their mother or father after 5 minutes of skin to skin with their mother. **Results:** Infants started to breastfeed significantly earlier if they had uninterrupted skin to skin with their mothers during the first 5 to 30 minutes. Skin to skin immediately after c-section enhances parental-infant interaction, uninterrupted skin to skin helps establish breastfeeding and lengthens the duration of breastfeeding even months after birth.

IN BRIEF

The best medical research and evidence supports skin to skin after c-section as long as mother and baby are healthy. The article listed above "The Natural Caesarean: A Woman Centred Technique" explains exactly how to achieve a c-section which enhances mother-baby bonding while maintaining a sterile OR.

Mother friendly hospitals such as Vanderbilt University Hospital in Tennessee are responding to their patients' desires to have immediate bonding and skin to skin with their baby in non-urgent, c-sections where baby and mother are healthy. Mothers and babies enjoy lifelong benefits from skin to skin including:

1. Earlier breastfeeding which leads to higher rates of success and longer duration.
2. Heart rate, respiration and body temperature more likely to be stable.

3. Less crying.
4. Beneficial increase in blood sugar.
5. Helps baby's motor system adjust.
6. Less anxiety for mom.
7. Less breast engorgement/pain 3 days after birth.

STEPS TO ASKING & PREPARING FOR SKIN TO SKIN
After C-Section:

1. Talk to your provider during your prenatal appointments about the fact that IF things should head in a C-section direction during labor that you'd like to do skin to skin ASAP after birth as long as all is well with mama and baby. If your provider says *"sure when you're in recovery"* then proceed to #2.

2. Politely let them know about the research you've been reading about no adverse effects and ask them to take a look at it, you can even print them out for them. (References are in the footnotes earlier in this chapter). And ask them to reconsider and set up another appointment where you can talk to the anesthesiologist and your provider together to come up with a plan of how to do this. Ask your anesthesiologist NOT to give you medications that are sedatives. You want to be as alert as possible. The remainder of the plan is below.

3. You'll need 2 support people in the operating room with you. One to help facilitate the skin to skin and the other to take pictures and help with baby. Doulas are a great help, and as you're interviewing, ask them about their experience facilitating skin to skin during C-sections.

4. Make sure you are wearing only your hospital gown (no bra, or camisole or anything underneath) and that your spouse or support is wearing a button down shirt so he can do skin to skin if needed.

5. Ask them to put the EKG leads on the sides of your body instead of on your chest, so that you can have space for baby with no interference from monitors.

6. Talk to your spouse and have them remind the nurses that instead of being brought to the warmer, if baby and mama are stable, they would like baby to be brought ASAP to mama. Since this is probably not standard operating procedure, it's important for dad or birth support to gently remind them.

7. While your partner meets your baby and is bringing baby to you, have your doula or other birth support get your gown unfastened and into skin to skin ready position. And make sure your support has a camera to take pics!

8. Ask if your hands can be unrestrained at this time, but even if they can't, continue. Have birth support help dad unswaddle baby and place horizontally across both mom's breasts, so baby and mama are chest to chest (and skin to skin), then have birth support cover mama and baby with blankets.

9. **One person must have their hands on baby at all times**, to make sure baby is secure on mama's chest. Baby will probably start rooting around lookin' for mama's booby. If possible, situate baby so she can find what she's lookin' for. Mama may also be able to use her hands to help with this and stroke and touch baby. All of the holding of baby in place is done by the spouse or birth support.

10. If mama starts feeling not well, have partner ready to take baby and do skin to skin instead. The button down shirt is handy here, and there will probably be scrubs to contend with as well which can be cut to make room for baby on the chest. Staying near mom while doing skin to skin is awesome, if possible.

11. Ask the nursing staff to wait until that golden hour (or two) is over before they weigh and measure baby.

TOP 5 PROVIDER OBJECTIONS
TO DELAYED CORD CLAMPING
AND HOW TO RESPOND

1. Your provider might say ... *"Delayed cord clamping takes too much time, my practice is just too busy."*

Your Response ... Nearly 1/3 of my baby's blood is still in the placenta and umbilical cord after birth. The benefits of:

- **Up to 33% more blood for my baby**
- **More red blood cells which carry oxygen to my baby's vital organs**
- **More white blood cells which fight off disease, bacteria & viruses**
- **More hematopoietic stem cells -strengthens immunity**
- **Less likelihood of anemia**
- **Awesome Iron stores through 6 months old improving brain development, etc. and the fact it will only take a few minutes. Don't you agree all these clinically measurable benefits for my baby's health are worth minutes of your time?**

2. *"Immediately clamping the cord prevents severe postpartum hemorrhage."*

Your Response: Actually, research doesn't support that. A 2009 Cochrane review[1] of 5 trials including 2,200 mamas found that there was no significant difference between early cord clamping and delayed cord clamping as far as postpartum hemorrhage or severe hemorrhage. You can check it out here.

---

[1] http://apps.who.int/rhl/reviews/CD004074sp.pdf

3. *"Healthy babies born at term don't get benefits from delayed cord clamping."*

Your Response: Studies don't show that to be the case at all. It doesn't matter when baby is born- they all receive the benefits of delayed cord clamping. In fact, babies that receive delayed cord clamping have a much easier time transitioning after birth and efficiently pumping blood to their organs and their lungs to breathe. Plus, the concentration of fetal stem cells is at an all-time high after birth. These stem cells help organ systems grow and develop. Depriving my baby of these beneficial stem cells *could* predispose him/her to diseases like chronic lung disease, asthma, diabetes, epilepsy, cerebral palsy, Parkinson's disease, infection and neoplasm.[2] *(the point here is that we're just beginning to understand ALL the benefits and there are no significant risks. This statement by any provider is simply not supported by any medical evidence.)*

4. *"Delayed cord clamping can lead to jaundice."*

Your Response: You are correct, studies show that there is an increased chance that delayed cord clamping will lead to jaundice. According to Mayo Clinic, treatment is often not even necessary for mild jaundice. Once the baby's liver gets acclimated and starts functioning fully (which will happen more effectively when delayed cord clamping delivers more oxygen and more blood to my baby's organs), it's no

---

[2] http://www.aimsusa.org/library/Tolosa%20-%20Cord%20Clamping%202009.12.04.pdf

problem. If the jaundice is more severe, light therapy and even putting baby in the sun for a few minutes each day will help. The benefits of delayed cord clamping far outweigh the potential risk for jaundice, according to the best research and evidence. Wouldn't you agree? [3]

5. *"You can't do delayed cord clamping and skin to skin because gravity will reduce the flow of blood from placenta to your baby."*

Your Response: You have a point, gravity is a factor. But the only influence gravity has is how long the placental transfusion actually takes. If baby is on my chest doing skin to skin, it may take longer for the placental transfusion to complete, but it will still happen. [4]

*The point here friends is that nothing your provider might say trumps what the best research evidence says. All of the research evidence says delayed cord clamping will help your baby in measurable ways. And unless there is some severe problem with baby (in which they need to operate right away, etc.), there is no reason why you can't have delayed cord clamping for your baby (even with a C-section, etc.)

---

[3] http://www.ncbi.nlm.nih.gov/pubmed/18425897
[4] http://www.ncbi.nlm.nih.gov/pubmed/22843002

HOW TO TALK TO YOUR PROVIDER ABOUT DELAYED CORD CLAMPING

"Excuse me Dr. _____, but I just read the latest evidence in the Journal of Pediatrics that it's best to delay cord clamping and that means I would like to receive my baby on my chest and keep my baby there for at least an hour. I'm sure that you would agree with me that this is the best thing for neurological development and the enhancement of breast feeding and bonding."

*If your provider pushes back on doing delayed cord clamping, you and your partner and birth support can let them know that you have spiritual intentions, you can say something like:

"Dr._____ or Nurse_____, we have a spiritual practice that is really important to us. Right after baby is born, we will need to have a spiritual moment (prayer time). Please respect this time and wait until we are done to proceed with whatever you need to do."

Or you can say:

"Dr. _____, this is a spiritual practice for me, I need to know that you support it. We would like for you to wait until we are finished with our prayer time before you do anything, including cutting the cord after baby is born. Please place our baby on my chest and give my partner and I, a couple moments. Thank you for respecting our beliefs."

The Pros & Cons of Cord Banking Blood

	PROS	CONS
Private Cord Blood Banking		
Public Cord Blood Banking		
Neither		

A couple questions to guide you:

1. What is the medical history in your family? Are there any known diseases that genetically you or a loved one could be susceptible to?
2. Will you feel a peace of mind?
3. How much is that peace of mind worth to you?

Questions to Ask Your Provider About Cord Blood Banking (private & public)

1. Do you recommend cord blood banking? Why?
2. Is the hospital where I will deliver, part of a public cord blood collection program?
3. What is your experience with private cord blood banking?
4. Do you recommend any specific bank?
    a. Why?
    b. Are you paid by these banks?
5. If we decide to do delayed cord clamping, and blood banking, do you see any problems with that?

Questions to Ask Private Cord Blood Banks

1. How is the cord blood collected?
2. What are your special techniques to assure that you get the most cord blood possible?
3. Is it possible to do delayed cord clamping and bank cord blood with your company?
   a. Why or why not?
4. What is the minimum amount of cord blood you will bank?
5. What if the collection is not suitable? How do we get our money back?
6. How much is collection & banking per year?
   a. Does the price change with the amount collected?
   b. Is there a guaranteed price on yearly storage? How long?
   c. Do you have any discounts or promotions?
7. How does the cord blood get from the hospital to your lab- where is your lab?
8. How can we be sure that the cord blood we donate, will not get mixed up with someone else's?
9. What security is in place to protect the cord blood while it is in the liquid nitrogen?
10. What about natural disasters? Do you have emergency plans in place?
11. Are you accredited? If so, with whom?
12. What process do we need to go through if we need to retrieve our cord blood?
13. What happens if we can't afford to pay for storage or we just decide we don't want to?
14. Can we tour your lab? (if we're in the area)
15. What assurances do we have that your company will still be here in 20 or 30 years?
16. In the event that the company folds, are we able to transfer our cord blood to another bank?
17. Do you have any guarantees?

Copyright

Sources

[i] http://www.cdc.gov/breastfeeding/data/mpinc/data/2009/tables1_1a-1_5a.htm

[ii] http://www.ideassonline.org/pdf/br_11_37.pdf

[iii] http://www.ncbi.nlm.nih.gov/pubmed/19489802

[iv] Haddad GG, Green TP. Diagnostic approach to respiratory disease. In: Kliegman RM,Behrman RE, Jenson HB, Stanton BF, eds.*Nelson Textbook of Pediatrics.*19th ed. Philadelphia, Pa: Saunders Elsevier; 2011:chap 366.

[v] Guarner F, Malagelada JR (February 2003). "Gut flora in health and disease". Lancet 361 (9356): 512–9. doi:10.1016/S0140-6736(03)12489-0.PMID 12583961.

[vi] http://www.nytimes.com/2013/05/19/magazine/say-hello-to-the-100-trillion-bacteria-that-make-up-your-microbiome.html?pagewanted=all&_r=3&

[vii] http://www.thelancet.com/journals/lancet/article/PIIS0140-6736(03)12489-0/fulltext

[viii] http://www.ncbi.nlm.nih.gov/pubmed/19489802

[ix] http://www.ncbi.nlm.nih.gov/pubmed/22592691

[x] http://summaries.cochrane.org/CD003519/early-skin-to-skin-contact-for-mothers-and-their-healthy-newborn-infants

[xi] http://pediatrics.aappublications.org/content/113/4/858.short

[xii] Affonso D, et al. Reconciliation and healing for mothers through skin-to-skin contact provided in an American tertiary level intensive care nursery. Neonatal Network, 1999,12:25-32

[xiii] http://yourbabybooty.com/ybb/wp-content/uploads/2013/11/Summary-of-Evidence-skin-to-skin.pdf

[xiv] http://www.ncbi.nlm.nih.gov/pubmed/22456657

[xv] Nolan, A., & Lawrence, C. (2009) A pilot study of a nursing intervention protocol to minimize maternal-infant separation after cesarean birth. Journal Obstetric, Gynecologic and Neonatal Nursing, 38(4), 430-442 DOI: 10.1111/j.1552-6909.2009.01039

[xvi] http://www.ncbi.nlm.nih.gov/pubmed/22456657

[xvii] http://www.ncbi.nlm.nih.gov/pubmed/21083718

[xviii] http://www.ncbi.nlm.nih.gov/pubmed/19614878

[xix] http://www.ncbi.nlm.nih.gov/pubmed/17542814

[xx] http://www.ncbi.nlm.nih.gov/pubmed/22077187

[xxi] http://summaries.cochrane.org/CD003519/early-skin-to-skin-contact-for-mothers-and-their-healthy-newborn-infants

[xxii] http://www.cdc.gov/breastfeeding/data/mpinc/data/2009/tables1_1b-1_5b.htm
[xxiii] http://www.cdc.gov/breastfeeding/data/mpinc/data/2009/tables1_1b-1_5b.htm
[xxiv] http://www.medscape.com/viewarticle/807746
[xxv]

http://onlinelibrary.wiley.com/doi/10.1002/14651858.CD004074.pub3/abstract
[xxvi] http://www.ncbi.nlm.nih.gov/pubmed/19022985
[xxvii] http://jama.jamanetwork.com/article.aspx?articleid=206143
[xxviii] http://www.aimsusa.org/library/Tolosa%20-%20Cord%20Clamping%202009.12.04.pdf
[xxix] http://informahealthcare.com/doi/abs/10.1080/01443610802712918
[xxx] http://cyclinginvestigation.usada.org/
[xxxi] http://www.mayoclinic.com/health/infant-jaundice/DS00107
[xxxii] http://www.thelancet.com/journals/lancet/article/PIIS0140-6736(12)60206-2/abstract
[xxxiii] http://cord-clamping.com/2011/09/05/who-optimal-timing-of-umbilical-cord-clamping/
[xxxiv] http://apps.who.int/rhl/reviews/CD004074sp.pdf
[xxxv] http://apps.who.int/rhl/reviews/CD004074sp.pdf
[xxxvi] http://www.aimsusa.org/library/Tolosa%20-%20Cord%20Clamping%202009.12.04.pdf
[xxxvii] http://www.ncbi.nlm.nih.gov/pubmed/18425897
[xxxviii] http://www.ncbi.nlm.nih.gov/pubmed/22843002
[xxxix] http://pediatrics.aappublications.org/content/123/3/1011.abstract
[xl] http://pediatrics.aappublications.org/content/123/3/1011.abstract
[xli] http://europepmc.org/abstract/MED/8205082
[xlii] http://www.ncbi.nlm.nih.gov/pubmed/9603182
[xliii]

http://www.haematologica.org/content/96/11/1700.full.pdf+html?sid=ea9f7ee9-135c-4236-8071-20806b5b7049
[xliv] http://www.ncbi.nlm.nih.gov/pubmed/20837328
[xlv] http://www.ncbi.nlm.nih.gov/pubmed/1983224
[xlvi] http://www.sciencedirect.com/science/article/pii/S0268960X00901383
[xlvii]

http://site1365706034.hospedagemdesites.ws/uploads/aparentado%20melhor.pdf
[xlviii] http://www.ncbi.nlm.nih.gov/pubmed/7616801
[xlix] http://pediatrics.aappublications.org/content/119/1/165.full
[l] http://www.acog.org/About_ACOG/News_Room/News_Releases/2008/ACOG_Revises_Opinion_on_Cord_Blood_Banking
[li] http://www.ncbi.nlm.nih.gov/pubmed/20630358

lii
http://www.ncbi.nlm.nih.gov/pubmed?term=lund%20AND%20south%20africa%20AND%20ophthalmia
liii http://www.ncbi.nlm.nih.gov/pubmed/7838190
liv
http://www.ncbi.nlm.nih.gov/pmc/articles/PMC1971807/pdf/brjcancer00216-0134.pdf

lv http://www.ncbi.nlm.nih.gov/pubmed/1421901
lvi http://www.scribd.com/doc/110302041/Anton-Sutor-Vit-K-Def-Bleeding-Jurnal
lvii http://www.ncbi.nlm.nih.gov/pubmed/8564900
lviii Von Kries R. Vitamin K prophylaxis – A useful public health measure? Paediatr Perinat Epidemiol 1992;6:7-13.
lix http://pediatrics.aappublications.org/content/91/5/1001.full.pdf+html

lx http://www.ncbi.nlm.nih.gov/pubmed/22619475
lxi http://www.ncbi.nlm.nih.gov/pubmed/8588159
lxii http://www.ncbi.nlm.nih.gov/pubmed/11034761

lxiii http://www.schattauer.de/en/magazine/subject-areas/journals-a-z/thrombosis-and-haemostasis/contents/archive/issue/896/manuscript/4792/download.html

lxiv http://onlinelibrary.wiley.com/doi/10.1046/j.1365-2141.1999.01104.x/full
lxv http://pediatrics.aappublications.org/content/91/5/1001.full.pdf+html
lxvi http://seer.cancer.gov/search?q=childhood+cancer
lxvii http://summaries.cochrane.org/CD002776/prophylactic-vitamin-k-for-vitamin-k-deficiency-bleeding-in-neonates